Course Manual

Second Edition

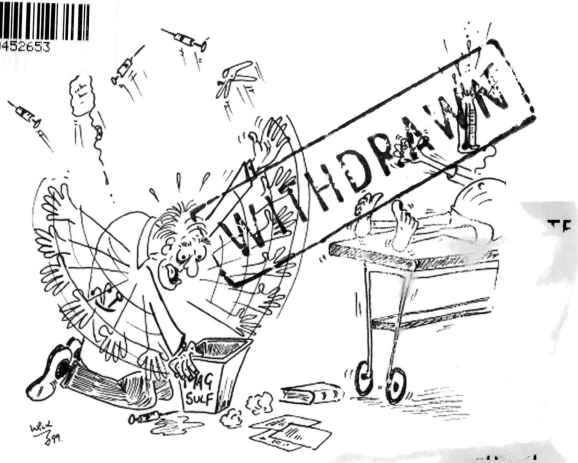

MAG
SULF

is allow.

Edited by

Cathy Winter, Jo Crofts, Chris Laxton,
Sonia Barnfield and Tim Draycott

PROMPT

PRactical Obstetric Multi-Professional Training

Practical locally based training
for obstetric emergencies

Course Manual

Edited by

Cathy Winter, Jo Crofts, Chris Laxton,
Sonia Barnfield and Tim Draycott

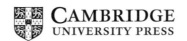

CAMBRIDGE
UNIVERSITY PRESS

University Printing House, Cambridge CB2 8BS, United Kingdom

Cambridge University Press is part of the University of Cambridge.

It furthers the University's mission by disseminating knowledge in the pursuit of education, learning and research at the highest international levels of excellence.

www.cambridge.org

© 2012 PROMPT Maternity Foundation

Registered Charity in England and Wales No. 1140557
Registered Company No. 7506593
Registered Office: Stone King LLP, 13 Queen Square, Bath, BA1 2HJ
www.promptmaternity.org

PROMPT Training Permissions and Licences
Units or institutions paying for a multi-professional team to attend an authorised PROMPT Train the Trainers (T3) Day are **only** permitted to run PROMPT multi-professional obstetric emergencies training courses, using PROMPT Course in a Box materials, within their own unit or institution.

Any PROMPT training conducted outside the unit or institution that has permission (see above) **requires a licence** from the PROMPT Maternity Foundation (PMF), e.g. a professional organisation or body wishing to roll out PROMPT training within a region or country, or a unit wishing to run PROMPT training at other hospitals outside of their own hospital group.

PMF are happy to discuss licensing arrangements or answer any questions relating to training permissions at any time. Please contact info@promptmaternity.org giving details of the training that is proposed.

First published 2008 by the Royal College of Obstetricians and Gynaecologists
This edition 2013 published by Cambridge University Press
5th printing 2015

Printed in the United Kingdom by Bell and Bain Ltd

A catalogue record for this publication is available from the British Library

ISBN   978-1-107-66052-6 Paperback

Cambridge University Press has no responsibility for the persistence or accuracy of URLs for external or third-party internet websites referred to in this publication, and does not guarantee that any content on such websites is, or will remain, accurate or appropriate.

....

Every effort has been made in preparing this book to provide accurate and up-to-date information which is in accord with accepted standards and practice at the time of publication. Although case histories are drawn from actual cases, every effort has been made to disguise the identities of the individuals involved. Nevertheless, the authors, editors and publishers can make no warranties that the information contained herein is totally free from error, not least because clinical standards are constantly changing through research and regulation. The authors, editors and publishers therefore disclaim all liability for direct or consequential damages resulting from the use of material contained in this book. Readers are strongly advised to pay careful attention to information provided by the manufacturer of any drugs or equipment that they plan to use.

Contents

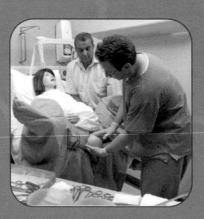
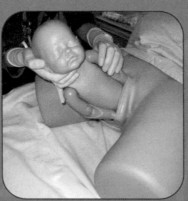
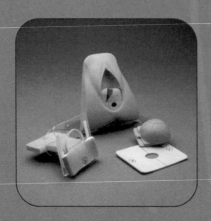

Contributors

Lt Col Tracy-Louise Appleyard	Consultant Obstetrician and Gynaecologist, Bristol/RAMC
Mr George Attilakos	Consultant Obstetrician, London
Dr Sonia Barnfield	Consultant Obstetrician, Bristol
Ms Christine Bartlett	Senior Midwife, Gloucester
Dr Joanna Crofts	Clinical Lecturer, University of Bristol
Dr Fiona Donald	Consultant Anaesthetist, Bristol
Professor Timothy Draycott	Consultant Obstetrician, Bristol
Dr Sian Edwards	Research Registrar, Bristol
Ms Denise Ellis	Senior Midwife, Bristol
Mr Christopher Eskell	PROMPT Maternity Foundation, Executive Member
Mr Robert Fox	Consultant Obstetrician, Taunton
Mr Simon Grant	Consultant Obstetrician, Bristol
Dr Judith Hyde	Consultant Obstetrician, Bristol
Mr Mark James	Consultant Obstetrician and Gynaecologist, Gloucester
Ms Sharon Jordan	Senior Midwife, Bristol
Dr Christina Laxton	Consultant Anaesthetist, Bristol
Ms Sharyn Mckenna	Maternity Risk Manager, Bristol
Dr Neil Muchatuta	Consultant Anaesthetist, Bristol
Dr Kate O'Brien	Specialty Registrar in Obstetrics & Gynaecology, Bristol
Dr David Odd	Consultant Neonatologist, Bristol
Ms Beverley Osborne	Senior Midwife, Bristol
Ms Helen Ping	Senior Midwife, Bristol

Dr Alison Pike · Consultant Neonatologist, Bristol

Dr Mark Scrutton · Consultant Anaesthetist, Bristol

Ms Debbie Senior · Practice Development Midwife, Bristol

Dr Dimitris Siassakos · Clinical Lecturer, University of Bristol

Mr Thabani Sibanda · Consultant Obstetrician, New Zealand

Dr Rebecca Simms · Research Registrar, Bristol

Ms Angie Sledge · Senior Midwife, Bristol

Dr Nicky Weale · Consultant Anaesthetist, Bristol

Ms Cathy Winter · PROMPT Maternity Foundation Midwife

Dr Anoushka Winton · Specialty Trainee in Anaesthesia

Ms Stephanie Withers · Labour Ward Matron, Bristol

Ms Heather Wilcox · Senior Midwife, Bristol

Ms Elaine Yard · Senior Midwife, Bristol

Mr Andy Yelland · Senior Midwife, Bristol

Ms Mandi Yelland · Senior Midwife, Bristol

Acknowledgements

The PROMPT Maternity Foundation (PMF) is a registered charity in England and Wales (Charity No. 1140557). The aim of the charity is to improve awareness and facilitate the distribution of effective obstetric emergencies training to areas of the world requesting access to an economical and sustainable training model. This is a significant project aimed at reducing maternal and perinatal morbidity and mortality.

This is the second edition of the PROMPT Course Manual. It has been developed and produced with the support of:

- Staff of North Bristol NHS Trust
- The South West Obstetric Network
- All researchers, facilitators and participants of the SaFE Study (Department of Health, UK)
- Limbs and Things, Bristol
- Laerdal Medical, Norway
- Ferring Pharmaceuticals, UK

The final production of the PROMPT Course in a Box would not have been possible without the invaluable help and support of:

- The Louise Stratton Memorial Fund
- Colstons Girls School, Bristol
- Mrs Lewis, Bristol
- Meg Winter, Bristol

PROMPT training is endorsed by:

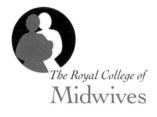

The Royal College of
Midwives

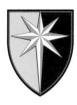

Royal College of
Obstetricians and Gynaecologists

Bringing to life the best in women's health care

Obstetric
Anaesthetists'
Association

List of abbreviations and terms

ABC ....airway, breathing, circulation

AED ....automated external defibrillator

ALS ....advanced life support

ALT.....................alanine aminotransferase

APH ....antepartum haemorrhage

APTT ....activated partial thromboplastin time

AST ....aspartate aminotransferase

AVPU ....alert, responsive to voice, responsive to painful stimuli or unresponsive

BP ....blood pressure

bpm ....beats/minute

Ca^{2+} ....calcium

CESDI..................Confidential Enquiry into Stillbirths and Deaths in Infancy

CMACE...............Centre for Maternal and Child Enquiries

CNST...................Clinical Negligence Scheme for Trusts

CO_2.....................carbon dioxide

CPR....................cardiopulmonary resuscitation

CT.......................computed tomography

CTG ....cardiotocograph

CTPA..................computed tomography pulmonary angiography

CVA ....cerebrovascular accident

CVP....................central venous pressure

DIC ....disseminated intravascular coagulation

ECG ....electrocardiogram

ECV....................external cephalic version

EFM ....electronic fetal heart rate monitoring

FBC ....full blood count

FFP ....fresh frozen plasma

HELLP syndrome..haemolysis, elevated liver enzymes and low platelets

HELP ....Head Elevating Laryngoscopy Pillow

HIE ....hypoxic ischaemic encephalopathy

HIV.....................human immunodeficiency virus

IM ....intramuscular

IPPV ....intermittent positive pressure ventilation

ITU ....intensive therapy unit

IV ....intravenous

K$^+$........................potassium

LFT ....liver function test

LMA...................laryngeal mask airway

MOEWS ....modified obstetric early warning score

MRI....................magnetic resonance imaging

Na$^+$......................sodium

NHSLA ....NHS Litigation Authority

NICE...................National Institute for Health and Clinical Excellence

NPSA..................National Patient Safety Agency

PaCO$_2$ ....arterial partial pressure of carbon dioxide

PaO$_2$....................arterial partial pressure of oxygen

PEA ....pulseless electrical activity

PPH ....postpartum haemorrhage

RCOG ....Royal College of Obstetricians and Gynaecologists

rFVIIa...................recombinant factor VIIa

SBAR...................situation, background, assessment and recommendation/response

U&Es ....urea and electrolytes

UKOSS ....United Kingdom Obstetric Surveillance System

VBAC ....vaginal birth after caesarean

VF ....ventricular fibrillation

VT ....ventricular tachycardia

WBC ....white blood cell count

WOMAN trial ......World Maternal Antifibrinolytic trial

Foreword

The world's attention is on the Millennium Development Goals (MDGs). MDG 4 aims to reduce child mortality, of which 50% are newborns, and MDG 5 aims to reduce maternal mortality. Pregnancy, labour and birth are in the most part safe, but some births are not as safe as they could or should be.

The research of the PROMPT Maternity Foundation and its members has confirmed that leadership and multi-professional teamworking, together with the appropriate knowledge and clinical skills, are essential to provide the best care for the mother and the fetus/newborn and thus to achieve MDGs 4 and 5. PROMPT provides just such training and has been associated with improvements in perinatal outcomes.

The PROMPT training package consists of a 'Course in a Box' which includes a Course Manual, a Trainer's Manual and a CD-ROM of lectures and videos. It provides course materials to enable local staff to run 'in-house' multi-professional obstetric emergencies courses in their own maternity units or other local settings.

The training package is written by a team of expert researchers who have many years of experience of conducting PROMPT training both locally and around the world. The evaluation of the effectiveness of the training with regard to its associated improvements in clinical outcomes is a priority of the PROMPT team. This scientific evidence is the hallmark of PROMPT.

Improving safety and quality by better knowledge, skills, teamwork and leadership is our responsibility. I am sure those who attend the PROMPT training programme and use the PROMPT materials will be able to deliver safe, high-quality care.

Sir Sabaratnam Arulkumaran
Professor and Head of Obstetrics and Gynaecology,
St George's, University of London   April 2012

Module 1
Teamworking

Key learning points

- To understand the importance of good team working.
- To understand that effective communication is vital in emergency situations.
- To understand the importance of stating the problem early.
- To appreciate the different roles and responsibilities of members of a multi-professional team.
- To understand the importance of shared decision making within the team.
- To recognise the value of being able to 'stand back and take a broader view' in an emergency situation – situational awareness.

Introduction

Obstetric emergencies are unpredictable and sudden. Successful management requires a rapid coordinated response by often ad hoc multi-professional teams. The need to provide training in team coordination and communication for clinicians has been repeatedly identified as a safety priority.

The most recent Centre for Maternal and Child Enquiries (CMACE) review reported that 70% of the direct maternal deaths could have been prevented with better care;[1] a lack of multi-professional team working and communication failures were once again identified as contributory factors.[2,3] Moreover, previous Confidential Enquires into Maternal Deaths in the United Kingdom have identified poor communication and poor team working as major contributors to fetal and neonatal mortality.[4,5] The Enquiries have recommended multi-professional obstetric emergencies

1

training, including teamwork training, for all staff providing care for mothers and babies.

The Clinical Negligence Scheme for Trusts (CNST) Maternity Clinical Risk Management Standards mandate that there should be a systematic process in maternity units for ensuring that multi-professional drill training is provided for all relevant obstetric and midwifery staff.[6] Similar recommendations have been made in the USA and Canada.[7]

CNST is an NHS Litigation Authority (NHSLA) insurance scheme for England and Wales by which maternity hospitals with a high standard of training, guidelines and audit are rewarded with reduced insurance premiums.

Definitions

Teamwork is the combined effective action of a group working towards a common goal. It requires individuals with different roles to communicate effectively and work together in a coordinated manner to achieve a successful outcome.

Teamwork training

Conventional healthcare training has typically focused on specific, technically skilled tasks. However, with the increasingly multi-professional nature of healthcare provision, focusing on individual theoretical knowledge, technical skills and attitude may be inadequate.[8] Multi-professional team training for obstetric emergencies has been associated with improved performance,[9] improved safety attitudes[10] and improved perinatal outcomes.[11,12]

Teamwork training recognises that people make fewer errors when they work in effective teams. Each member of the team can understand their responsibilities when processes are planned and standardised, with team members 'looking out' for one another and trapping errors before they cause an accident.[13]

There is also evidence that, even when training is conducted in multi-professional teams, some clinical teams possess characteristics that make them more efficient than others, and they are better able to achieve good outcomes by performing key actions in a timely manner. However, these characteristics are not explained by differences in knowledge or skill,[8] emphasising that training needs to include other aspects of team working.

Improvements in outcomes

As previously mentioned, current evidence supports training for obstetric emergencies in multi-professional teams, the most notable evidence being the association between improved obstetric and perinatal outcomes after clinical training with integrated teamwork training.[14] However, not all training is equal, and some training programmes have increased the rate of poor perinatal outcomes rather than improving them.[15] Also, teamwork training in isolation has not proved to be effective in obstetrics.[16,17]

The key features of training programmes associated with improvements in perinatal outcome are:[14,17]

- training is conducted in-house
- 100% of maternity staff are trained regularly
- all maternity staff are trained together, incorporating teamwork principles into clinical training scenarios
- system changes are introduced, often suggested by staff after participating in the training.

In-house training appears to be the most efficient and cost-effective means of training all staff in an institution. In-house training can also address specific local issues and can be used as a driver for system changes.[10,14,18] Moreover, training within the local environment may be the most effective way of improving outcomes.[19]

Finally, in one obstetric study, it was found that more efficient teams were likely to have stated (recognised and verbally declared) the emergency earlier, and to have managed the critical task using closed-loop communication (task clearly and loudly delegated, accepted, executed and completion acknowledged). Such teams were noted to have administered magnesium sulphate within the allocated time (10 minutes), had significantly fewer exits from the labour room and used a structured form of communication.[20] It is vital that these communication skills are integrated into clinical training.

Communication

Communication is the transfer of information and the sharing of meaning. Often, the purpose of communication is to clarify or acknowledge the receipt of the information. Communication is often impaired under stress. It is important to learn effective techniques that increase awareness and help overcome these limitations.

The five requirements for effective communication and efficient team performance are:[21,22]

1. **FORMULATED**

   Give a clear message. It should be succinct and not rambling. SBAR (situation, background, assessment and recommendation/response) is a useful acronym for formulating messages and handing over information[20] and was used almost naturally by the most effective obstetric teams.[9,20] For example:

   > 'Jenny James is unwell with sepsis (S). She is 33 weeks pregnant and her membranes ruptured 1 week ago (B). She is in pain, is hypotensive and tachycardic, and her observations score 3 on the MOEWS chart (A). I would like a senior obstetrician and senior midwife to review her immediately (R).'

   Figure 1.1 is an example of a maternal SBAR form that may be used when handing over information.

2. **ADDRESSED TO SPECIFIC INDIVIDUALS (DELEGATED)**

   Use names of staff, and/or establish visual contact. Allocate appropriate tasks to an identified recipient.

   > 'Liz and Susan (midwives), please can you help get Mrs Jones into McRoberts' position.'

   > 'Hazel (maternity healthcare assistant), please could you document times and actions as they are called out, on this laminated pro forma. Thanks.'

3. **DELIVERED**

   The message should be sent clearly, concisely and calmly. When the obstetric emergency team arrives in your room, say:

   > 'Susan Jones is having a postpartum haemorrhage. She has lost approximately one litre of blood. Her placenta has been delivered and appears complete, and she has an intact perineum. I have given her one dose of IM Syntometrine but her uterus still feels atonic.'

SBAR report to clinician about a clinical obstetric situation

S | **Situation**

I am calling about (woman's name): _____ Ward: _____ Hosp No: _____

The problem I am calling about is: _____
I have just made an assessment:

The vital signs are: Blood pressure ____ / ____ Pulse ____ Respirations ____ SPO$_2$ ____ % Temperature ____ ^{0}C

I am concerned about:
  Blood pressure because it is:
    systolic over 160
    diastolic over 100
    systolic less than 90
  Pulse because it is:
    over 120
    less than 40
  Respirations because they are:
    less than 10
    over 30
    The woman is having oxygen at
    _____ l/min
  Maternal temperature because it is: ____ ^{0}C

  Maternal serum lactate because it is: _____ mmol/l

  Urine output because it is:
    less than 100mls over the last 4 hours
    significantly proteinuric (+++)
  Haemorrhage:
    Antepartum
    Postpartum
  Fetal wellbeing:
    Pathological CTG
  FBS Result: pH _____
    Time sample taken: _____ hrs

  Obstetric Early Warning Chart Score: [ ] [ ]

B | **Background** (tick relevant sections)
The woman is:
    Primparous   Multiparous   Grand multparous
    Gestation: _____ wks   Singleton   Multiple
    Previous Caesarean section or uterine surgery
Fetal wellbeing
    Abdominal palpation:
    Fundal height: ____cms   Presentation: _____ Fifths palpable: _____ FH rate: ____bpm
    CTG: Normal   Suspicious   Pathological
Antenatal
    A/N problem (details): _____
Labour
    Spontaneous onset   Induced
    IUGR   Pre eclampsia   Reduced Fetal movements   Diabetes   APH
    Syntocinon
    Most recent vaginal examination: Time _____hrs
    Cervical dilatation: _____cms   Station of presenting part: _____   Position: _____
    Membranes intact   Meconium stained liquor   Fresh red loss PV
    Third stage complete   Retained placenta
Postnatal
    Delivery date: _____ Delivery time: _____hrs
    Type of delivery: _____ Perineal trauma: _____
    Blood loss: _____mls   Syntocinon infusion
    Fundus: High   Atonic   Uterus tender   Abdominal/perineal wound oozing

    Treatment given / in progress: _____

A | **Assessment**
    I think the problem is: _____

    I am not sure what the problem is but the woman is deteriorating and we need to do something

R | **Recommendation**
    Request:
      Please come to see the woman immediately
      I think delivering needs to be expedited
      I think the woman needs to be transferred to delivery suite
      I would like advice please
    Reported to: _____   **Response:** _____

Person completing form (name): _____Date: _____ Time: _____

SBAR Clinical Obstetric reporting sheet. Please photocopy form and file original in woman's notes and copy with Risk Incident form

Figure 1.1 Example SBAR handover sheet

rather than:

> 'Oh dear, Susan has just had a really big baby and I gave her Syntometrine but she is bleeding, really, really heavily. Oh dear, please can someone help me.'

4. **ACKNOWLEDGED**
Adequate volume used and repeated back:

> 'You would like me to give a second dose of Syntometrine intramuscularly straight away?'

5. **ACTED UPON**
Meaning acknowledged and action performed:

> 'OK. That's one ampoule of Syntometrine given intramuscularly at 15:30.'

In addition, the use of non-verbal communication, including making eye contact with individuals, helps to prevent ambiguity and promotes a shared knowledge of intention. Improper terminology, inaudible communication, excess chatter and incomplete reports should be avoided.

Leadership: roles and responsibilities

Team leadership involves providing direction, structure and support for other team members. The team leader is often the most senior obstetrician present,[22] but may be the midwifery coordinator or anaesthetist – whoever knows the team members' roles and responsibilities and has adequate experience to anticipate the possible end to an emergency.[22] It is essential that the team leader is nominated, declared verbally and accepted by the rest of the team as early as possible.[22]

Team leaders vary in their level of expertise when involved in a particular emergency situation and also in their readiness to lead. The team leader requires a certain level of competence; however, it is unlikely that they will possess all the abilities of every team member present. Therefore, the team leader's role should be to coordinate the activities of the specialists within the team by communicating clearly and simply, delegating tasks appropriately and planning ahead.[22] In addition, a good team leader respects the expertise of each team member, is willing to listen and is open to criticism and constructive feedback.[22]

Other members of the team should have their individual roles identified and agreed as early as possible. The leader should allocate critical tasks to the team members, including a designated person to talk to the woman and her family.[22,23] Team members should be mutually supportive, communicate clearly and give regular updates. They should avoid becoming fixated on minutiae or running around aimlessly.[20]

Situational awareness: the bigger picture

Situational awareness is how we notice, understand and think ahead in a fast-paced, constantly changing situation. It is that 'gut instinct' or 'sixth sense' that makes an expert midwife, obstetrician or anaesthetist. It involves recognising and understanding important cues, anticipating problems and sharing them with the team so that shared decision making and goals are achieved.

Three levels of situational awareness have been suggested.[24] These levels are listed below and include examples related to obstetric emergencies.

1. **NOTICE**
   Be aware of the patient's status, the team members' status and all available resources; anticipate potential errors by noticing cues and sharing decision making:

   > 'The labour ward coordinator and the senior obstetrician on call are reviewing the labour ward board, as the labour ward is full and two of the women are very ill: one has severe pre-eclampsia and poor urine output and the other has had a 1000 ml postpartum haemorrhage and requires an examination under anaesthesia. In such circumstances, it is vital that both the midwifery and obstetric lead for the shift have an awareness of the serious problems that may develop. They can then anticipate and plan how to manage the cases and also consider which team members may be required to assist with the problems.'

2. **UNDERSTAND**
   Share information with the team, think what these cues and clues may mean, be aware of common pitfalls, re-evaluate/stand back at regular intervals, seek to engage other team members in decisions.

'On review of all the cases on the labour ward, the midwife coordinator and the senior obstetrician identify that there are several complicated problems that need decisions and action. They are considering whether it may be wise to call in the consultant obstetrician and anaesthetist for support and to assist with the management of these problematic cases. Before they can make this decision, both the midwife and the senior obstetrician go to each room for a thorough review, requesting an update from each of the midwives providing care. They then seek the opinion of the on-call anaesthetist to gain further information that may influence the actions to be taken.'

3. **THINK AHEAD**
   Anticipate, plan and prioritise:

   'Having sought further information and also the opinion of other team members, the labour ward coordinator and the senior obstetrician are now able to identify potential problems and therefore prioritise the cases to formulate an action plan. Their ability to do this is based not only upon the information provided by the other team members but also on their own knowledge and previous experience. In this instance, they both agree that their first action should be to call in the obstetric consultant for support and guidance in the management of the complicated cases.'

Situational awareness allows individuals to be 'ahead of the game'. Experienced clinicians usually have good situational awareness; they often pick up subtle cues, understand their significance and use them to anticipate and pre-empt problems.[22]

Recognising cues for loss of situational awareness

In extreme situations, people can sometimes enter 'fast time', whereby their capacity to reason is so severely impaired by the stress of the workload that they are no longer able to function interactively with the rest of the team.

Characteristic signs of 'fast time' include:

- poor communication
- inability to plan ahead
- tunnel vision
- fixation on irrelevant issues (such as less than ideal equipment) or displacement activities such as unnecessary disputes with colleagues.

'Fast time' at its worst can cause even good team players to completely 'freeze up'.

Maintaining/regaining situational awareness

One suggested way of maintaining situational awareness is to adopt the philosophy of the 'non-participant' leader: try not to become engaged in practical tasks that can be undertaken by others. This allows the leader to take a step back and maintain a broader view of the unfolding crisis. Team leaders sometimes have difficulty doing this in practice because they often have the particular 'hands on' skills required to deal with the problem.

To regain control of a situation, the following strategies should be tried:

- Take the 'helicopter view': stand back to get the bigger picture.[22]
- Declare an emergency early: you will engage everyone's attention and boost the available human resources. Early declaration is associated with improved clinical team performance and efficiency[20] but also with improved patient perception of care.[23]
- Communicate clearly and simply, starting with the critical tasks for each emergency.[23]
- Plan ahead: for example, prepare for a perimortem caesarean section early in cases of maternal collapse.
- Delegate the critical tasks appropriately.[20]

Team working under pressure

Pressure situations give us the feeling that everything needs to be done immediately and so the tendency to rush increases. Rushing tasks while under pressure increases the potential for making errors. Therefore, a good team leader should try to manage the emergency at a steady but efficient pace.

What makes a good team member?

- Good communicator
- Good understanding and acceptance of own limitations
- Awareness of environment and limitations of others
- Assertive
- Non-confrontational but willing to challenge if necessary
- Receptive to the suggestions of all other team members
- Thinks clearly

Key points

- Good team working is important because poorly functioning teams are associated with patient harm.
- More efficient teams state the emergency earlier and use closed-loop communication.
- Teamwork training may improve clinical outcomes when incorporated into clinical training.
- Multi-professional training locally for all staff has been associated with improved teamwork, improved safety attitudes and, most importantly, improved perinatal outcomes.

References

1.   Centre for Maternal and Child Enquiries. Saving Mothers' Lives: reviewing maternal deaths to make motherhood safer: 2006–08. *BJOG* 2011;118 Suppl 1:1–203.

2.   Lewis G (editor). The Confidential Enquiry into Maternal and Child Health (CEMACH). *Saving Mothers' Lives: Reviewing Maternal Deaths to Make Motherhood Safer 2003–2005. The Seventh Report on Confidential Enquiries into Maternal Deaths in the United Kingdom.* London: CEMACH; 2007.

3.   Lewis G (editor). The Confidential Enquiry into Maternal and Child Health (CEMACH). *Why Mothers Die 2000–2002. The Sixth Report on Confidential Enquiries into Maternal Deaths in the United Kingdom.* London: RCOG Press; 2004.

4.   Maternal and Child Health Research Consortium. *Confidential Enquiry into Stillbirths and Deaths in Infancy: 5th Annual Report, 1 January–31 December 1996.* London: Maternal and Child Health Research Consortium; 1998.

5.   Maternal and Child Health Research Consortium. *Confidential Enquiry into Stillbirths and Deaths in Infancy: 7th Annual Report, 1 January–31 December 1998.* London: Maternal and Child Health Research Consortium; 2000.

6.   NHS Litigation Authority. Clinical Negligence Scheme for Trusts Maternity Clinical Risk Management Standards. London: NHSLA; 2011 [http://www.nhsla.com/RiskManagement/].

7.   Sentinel event alert issue 30 July 21, 2004. Preventing infant death and injury during delivery. *Adv Neonatal Care* 2004;4:180–1.

8.   Siassakos D, Draycott TJ, Crofts JF, Hunt LP, Winter C, Fox R. More to teamwork than knowledge, skill and attitude. *BJOG* 2010;117:1262–9.

9.   Siassakos D, Fox R, Crofts JF, Hunt LP, Winter C, Draycott TJ. The management of a simulated emergency: better teamwork, better performance. *Resuscitation* 2011;82:203–6.

10. Siassakos D, Fox R, Hunt L, Farey J, Laxton C, Winter C, et al. Attitudes toward safety and teamwork in a maternity unit with embedded team training. *Am J Med Qual* 2011;26:132–7.

11. Draycott T, Sibanda T, Owen L, Akande V, Winter C, Reading S, et al. Does training in obstetric emergencies improve neonatal outcome? *BJOG* 2006;113:177–82.

12. Draycott TJ, Crofts JF, Ash JP, Wilson LV, Yard E, Sibanda T, et al. Improving neonatal outcome through practical shoulder dystocia training. *Obstet Gynecol* 2008;112:14–20.

13. Helmreich RL. On error management: lessons from aviation. *BMJ* 2000;320:781–5.

14. Siassakos D, Crofts JF, Winter C, Weiner CP, Draycott TJ. The active components of effective training in obstetric emergencies. *BJOG* 2009;116:1028–32.

15. MacKenzie IZ, Shah M, Lean K, Dutton S, Newdick H, Tucker DE. Management of shoulder dystocia: trends in incidence and maternal and neonatal morbidity. *Obstet Gynecol* 2007;110:1059–68.

16. Nielsen PE, Goldman MB, Mann S, Shapiro DE, Marcus RG, Pratt SD, et al. Effects of teamwork training on adverse outcomes and process of care in labor and delivery: a randomized controlled trial. *Obstet Gynecol* 2007;109:48–55.

17. Riley W, Davis S, Miller K, Hansen H, Sainfort F, Sweet R. Didactic and simulation nontechnical skills team training to improve perinatal patient outcomes in a community hospital. *Jt Comm J Qual Patient Saf* 2011;37:357–64.

18. Thompson S, Neal S, Clark V. Clinical risk management in obstetrics: eclampsia drills. *Qual Saf Health Care* 2004;13:127–9.

19. Siassakos D, Crofts J, Winter C, Draycott T; on behalf of the SaFE Study Group. Multi-professional 'fire-drill' training in the labour ward. *The Obstetrician & Gynaecologist* 2009;11:55–60.

20. Siassakos D, Bristowe K, Draycott TJ, Angouri J, Hambly H, Winter C, et al. Clinical efficiency in a simulated emergency and relationship to team behaviours: a multisite cross-sectional study. *BJOG* 2011;118:596–607.

21. Siassakos D, Draycott T, Montague I, Harris M. Content analysis of team communication in an obstetric emergency scenario. *J Obstet Gynaecol* 2009;29:499–503.

22. Bristowe K, et al., Leadership and teamwork for clinical emergencies: multisite interprofessional focus group analysis. Bristol: University of Bristol and University of the West of England; 2011.

23. Siassakos D, Bristowe K, Hambly H, Angouri J, Crofts JF, Winter C, et al. Team communication with patient actors: findings from a multisite simulation study. *Simul Healthc* 2011;6:143–9.

24. Endsley MR. The role of situation awareness in naturalistic decision making. In: Zsambok CE, Klein G (editors). *Naturalistic Decision Making*. New Jersey, USA: Lawrence Erlbaum Associates; 1997. p. 269–83.

Module 2
Basic life support and maternal collapse

Key learning points

- Assessment and resuscitation of maternal collapse:
  - ☐ A B C
  - ☐ Manual left uterine displacement or 30-degree left tilt if on firm tilting surface (e.g. operating table) to reduce aortocaval compression.
- Calling for help: effective communication of problem to team.
- Equipment: knowing where to find emergency trolley, defibrillator, anaphylaxis box.
- Appropriate documentation.

Common difficulties observed in training drills

- Failure to recognise cardiac arrest in a deteriorating patient.
- Not starting basic life support.
- Forgetting to keep woman supine with manual left uterine displacement.
- Not administering high-flow oxygen to mother.

Introduction

Maternal collapse occurs in a variety of circumstances. Presentation may range from an isolated and temporary drop in blood pressure to cardiac arrest and death. It is absolutely imperative that all healthcare professionals can provide basic resuscitation, regardless of the cause. In the 2007 CEMACH report,[1] resuscitation skills were considered poor in an unacceptably high number of the maternal deaths. This and the 2011 CMACE report[2] recommend that all clinical staff should undertake regular training to improve basic, intermediate and advanced life support skills.

Basic life support algorithm

All healthcare professionals should be aware of the principles of basic life support. An outline of the basic life support algorithm is provided in Figure 2.1, but it is not intended to be a complete guide. Further information is available from the Resuscitation Council (UK).[3]

What do we mean by maternal collapse?

Maternal collapse is severe respiratory or circulatory distress that may lead to a sudden change in level of consciousness or cardiac arrest if untreated. Any of the vital observations in Box 2.1 should trigger an emergency response.

Box 2.1 Observations that trigger an emergency response	
Airway	Obstructed or noisy
Breathing	Respiratory rate less than 5 or more than 35 breaths/minute
Circulation	Pulse rate less than 40 or more than 140 beats/minute
	Systolic blood pressure less than 80 or more than 180 mmHg
Neurology	Sudden decrease in level of consciousness
	Unresponsive or responsive to painful stimuli only
	Seizures

Figure 2.2 illustrates a systematic way of classifying possible causes of maternal collapse. The causes are discussed in more detail in the following sections.

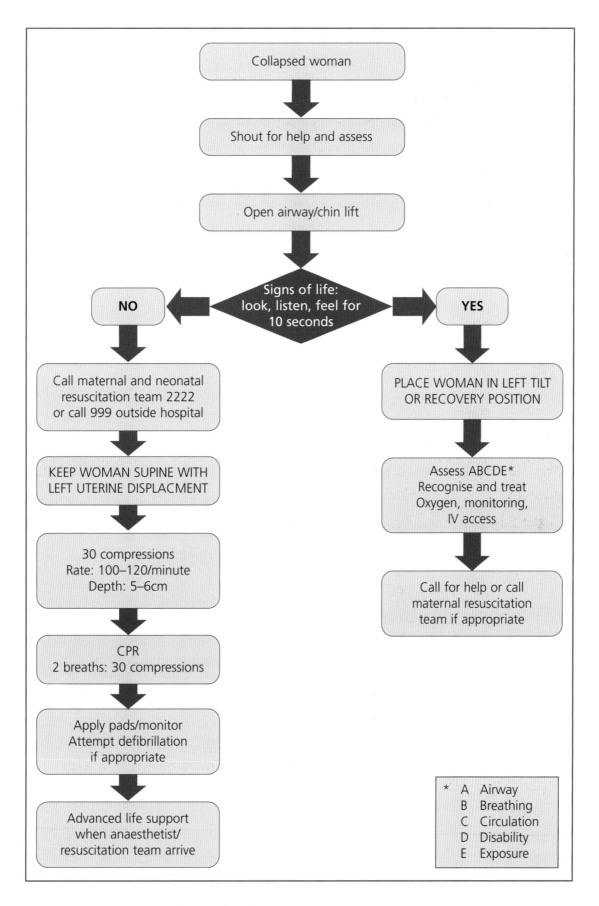

Figure 2.1 Basic life support algorithm

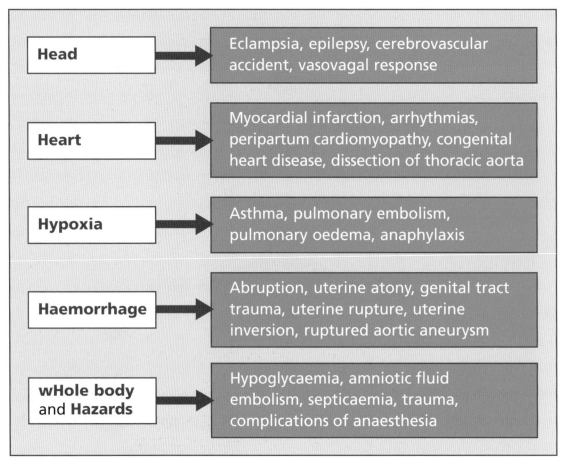

Head	Eclampsia, epilepsy, cerebrovascular accident, vasovagal response
Heart	Myocardial infarction, arrhythmias, peripartum cardiomyopathy, congenital heart disease, dissection of thoracic aorta
Hypoxia	Asthma, pulmonary embolism, pulmonary oedema, anaphylaxis
Haemorrhage	Abruption, uterine atony, genital tract trauma, uterine rupture, uterine inversion, ruptured aortic aneurysm
wHole body and **Hazards**	Hypoglycaemia, amniotic fluid embolism, septicaemia, trauma, complications of anaesthesia

Figure 2.2 Possible causes of maternal collapse

Management of maternal collapse

The key to the effective management of maternal collapse is a simple and structured approach to diagnosis and treatment. The underlying principles of the management of any critically ill patient are the same and are often described through the ABC approach (airway, breathing, circulation).

Initial management

- Assess the responsiveness of the woman by gently shaking her and asking if she is all right. If there is no response, seek immediate help using the emergency bell, dialling 2222 in hospital or 999 if outside hospital.

- Turn her on to her back and ask an assistant to manually displace the uterus to the left using one or two hands to reduce aortocaval obstruction (see Figure 3.1, page 27). A 30-degree tilt may be used if the woman is on a firm surface that can be tilted (e.g. operating table).

- Open the airway using head tilt and chin lift manoeuvres.

- Assess breathing by looking at movement of the chest wall, listening for breath sounds and feeling for air on your cheek (look, listen, feel) for up to 10 seconds. Agonal gasps (isolated or infrequent gasping in the absence of other breathing in an unconscious person) occur commonly in the first few minutes after sudden cardiac arrest; they are an indication for starting cardiopulmonary resuscitation (CPR) immediately and should not be confused with normal breathing.

- While assessing breathing, observe for other signs of life, such as colour and movement.

- If there are no signs of life, commence basic life support (Figure 2.1) until help arrives (to provide advanced life support) or the woman shows signs of life.

- If the woman has signs of life, place her in the recovery position and give high-flow oxygen via a reservoir mask. Obtain intravenous access, take blood samples (full blood count, clotting screen, urea and electrolytes, glucose, liver function tests, group and save) and give intravenous fluids. Establish monitoring of vital signs with electro-cardiogram (ECG), respirations, pulse, blood pressure measurement and pulse oximetry. Then perform a primary obstetric survey.

Primary obstetric survey

A primary obstetric survey should be performed in a logical manner, starting at the head and working downwards. This initial management should produce a working diagnosis and should enable treatment of the cause to commence. Box 2.2 shows the questions to be considered when performing the primary obstetric survey. It is important that senior obstetric and anaesthetic support is sought if not already present.

Decide on continuing treatment

After the primary survey, the cause of the collapse and treatment required may be evident; for example, eclampsia or haemorrhage. If the cause is not obvious, only a few key treatment decisions are necessary.

1. Is fluid resuscitation a priority or is it contraindicated? If in doubt, fluid is usually beneficial: the exception is when the woman has, or is at great risk of, pulmonary oedema, as may happen in severe pre-eclampsia or renal failure.

Box 2.2 Primary obstetric survey	
Head	How responsive is the patient? Is she alert, responsive to voice, responsive to painful stimuli or unresponsive (AVPU)? Is the patient fitting?
Heart	What is the capillary refill like? What is the pulse rate and rhythm? Is there a murmur?
Chest	Is there good bilateral air entry? What are the breath sounds like? Is the trachea central?
Abdomen	Is there an 'acute' abdomen (rebound and guarding)? Is there tenderness (uterine or non-uterine)? Is the fetus alive? Is there a need for a laparotomy or delivery?
Vagina	Is there bleeding? What is the stage of labour? Is there an inverted uterus?

2. Is a laparotomy required for diagnosis or treatment? Is there evidence of an acute abdominal event? Does the fetus need delivery to aid resuscitation?

3. Is sepsis likely and are antibiotics therefore a priority?

4. Is intensive care needed to provide airway, respiratory or circulatory support?

Secondary obstetric survey

Further management is dependent upon the cause of the collapse. Once the woman has been stabilised, a secondary obstetric survey should be performed (Box 2.3).

Box 2.3 Secondary obstetric survey	
ACTION	DETAIL
History	Revisit the history of the collapse and the previous history of the woman
	Read the notes and ask the partner or relatives
Examine	Repeat the examination going from top to toe
Investigate	Take arterial blood gases, troponins, blood glucose, lactate, blood cultures, ECG, chest X-ray, ultrasound of the abdomen and high vaginal swab
Monitor	Continue monitoring of ECG, respirations, pulse, blood pressure and pulse oximetry
	Consider arterial and central venous pressure lines to aid monitoring
Pause and think further	Consider further investigations such as CT/MRI scans and echocardiography
	Ask relevant experts for their opinions

Further key treatment decisions

Re-evaluate and continue to support the airway, breathing and circulation of the woman. Do you need intensive care to support?

Re-evaluate your working diagnosis at intervals to ensure the pattern still fits and treatment is working.

Specific causes of maternal collapse

Pulmonary thromboembolism

Pulmonary emboli are more common in pregnancy and the postpartum period, owing to the procoagulant effect of pregnancy and the mechanical obstruction by the abdominal uterus of venous return from the lower body. Pulmonary emboli may be small and non-symptomatic or large and cause instant collapse and rapid death. Thromboembolism remains a common cause of direct maternal death in the UK, with a rate of 0.79/100 000 maternities.[2]

Pulmonary emboli may present with shortness of breath, pleuritic chest pain, haemoptysis or sudden collapse in a woman who may or may not have signs of a deep vein thrombosis. Clinical signs may include tachycardia, tachypnoea, hypoxia and evidence of right heart strain on ECG (S1,Q3,T3) with a raised jugular venous pressure. Diagnosis can be difficult; initial assessment and treatment should be made on symptoms and signs plus arterial blood gases, ECG and chest X-ray, with the diagnosis confirmed by ventilation–perfusion scanning (VQ scan) or computed tomography pulmonary angiography (CTPA).

Treatment should be supportive using facial oxygen, with ventilatory and cardiovascular support as necessary. Anticoagulation with heparin (subcutaneous low-molecular-weight heparin or intravenous heparin) should be commenced on clinical suspicion of pulmonary embolism until the diagnosis is confirmed or refuted.

Haemorrhagic shock

Hypovolaemia, usually secondary to haemorrhage, is the most common cause of shock in obstetric patients. Signs of hypovolaemia include:

- tachycardia and tachypnoea
- cold, pale skin
- hypotension
- reduced urine output
- altered level of consciousness
- narrowed pulse pressure (less than 35 mmHg difference between systolic and diastolic readings).

Prompt resuscitative fluid replacement is essential. If there is significant haemorrhage, arterial and central venous pressure (CVP) lines are often useful adjuncts for monitoring. The cause is most commonly obstetric in nature (such as uterine atony, abruption, ruptured uterus), but non-obstetric causes should also be considered.

Although rare, aneurysm rupture may occur (such as aortic, renal, splenic, iliac). This is often not recognised but is identified as a cause of maternal mortality in the Confidential Enquiries.[1] Urgent laparotomy should be considered when there are signs of an acute abdomen in conjunction with hypovolaemia.

Eclamptic seizures and coma

Eclamptic seizures and coma may resemble amniotic fluid embolus syndrome, but the presence of hypertension, proteinuria and oedema in the eclamptic woman differentiates these two conditions. For more information about diagnosis and treatment, refer to **Module 6**.

Cerebrovascular accident

Cerebrovascular accidents (CVAs) can present with any manner of neurological signs. CVAs can be embolic or haemorrhagic in origin. Raised blood pressure, for example in severe pre-eclampsia, is a risk factor for CVA and any pregnant woman with systolic blood pressure of 160 mmHg or greater requires antihypertensive treatment to reduce the risk of a CVA.[1] Migrainous attacks can mimic CVAs. A CT or magnetic resonance imaging (MRI) scan should aid in diagnosis and direct treatment.

Septicaemic shock

Maternal sepsis was the leading cause of death in the 2006–2008 triennium.[2] It is crucially important that the symptoms and signs are recognised and acted upon directly. For more information about diagnosis and treatment, refer to **Module 7**.

Disseminated intravascular coagulation

Disseminated intravascular coagulation (DIC) can occur secondary to massive bleeding, severe infection, amniotic fluid embolism or anaphylaxis. When DIC occurs, there is an excessive consumption of platelets and clotting factors, resulting in a prolonged clotting time, low platelets, low fibrinogen and haemorrhage. Spontaneous bleeding may be noticed from needle puncture, intravenous cannulae or epidural sites. Vaginal haemorrhage may also occur, as may bleeding from the woman's gums.

Early involvement of haematology, senior obstetric and anaesthetic staff, as well as intensive care, is vital if DIC is suspected. Blood should be sent for full blood count, cross-matching, clotting, fibrinogen and D-dimers. Haematology should advise on the appropriate blood products required to correct clotting. The cause of DIC should be investigated promptly and treated appropriately.

Hypo- or hyperglycaemia

Women with diabetes may collapse into a hypoglycaemic coma. Although rare, type 1 diabetes mellitus may commence in pregnancy. Blood glucose should always be tested in a collapsed or fitting woman if the cause is not obvious, and urine should be tested for the presence of ketones if diabetic ketoacidosis is suspected. Acute fatty liver may also present with maternal hypoglycaemia. If blood glucose is found to be below 3 mmol/l, 50 ml of 20% glucose solution should be administered intravenously.

Acute heart failure

Cardiac disease is the most common cause of indirect maternal death, as well as the most frequent cause of maternal death overall.[1,2] A known history of cardiac disease, chest pain with ECG changes or a new cardiac murmur may help to establish the diagnosis. If chest pain is a presenting feature, troponin levels should be taken 6 hours after the onset of pain. If cardiac ischaemia is suspected, 300 mg aspirin should be given orally unless contraindicated. If cardiac failure is suspected or there is a new murmur on auscultation, urgent senior medical review and echocardiography should be arranged.

Pulmonary aspiration of gastric contents

Pregnancy increases the risk of pulmonary aspiration of gastric contents. This is because of progesterone-induced relaxation of the oesophageal sphincter and delayed stomach emptying, a problem which becomes more pronounced during labour. Aspiration is most likely to occur in the unconscious obstetric patient (for example, during induction or emergence from general anaesthesia) owing to the loss of the cough reflex. Gastric aspiration may present with coughing, cyanosis, tachypnoea, tachycardia, hypotension or pulmonary oedema.

Anaphylactic or toxic reaction to drugs or allergens

Anaphylactic or toxic reaction to drugs or allergens may present as convulsions or collapse. The close timing of administration of the drug or allergen (such as latex) in relation to the collapse may be indicative of an anaphylactoid or toxic reaction.

Severe anaphylaxis should be treated with:

■ oxygen 100% via mask with reservoir bag

■ adrenaline (epinephrine) 500 micrograms (0.5 ml of 1:1000) IM (into side of thigh), repeated every 5 minutes if necessary

■ **OR** if an anaesthetist is present, up to 1 mg IV adrenaline (epinephrine) at a concentration of 1 in 10 000; adrenaline (epinephrine) should be diluted to a concentration of 100 micrograms/ml (1 mg in 10 ml) and then given in 0.5 ml aliquots as required

■ prepare other drugs: chlorphenamine 10 mg IV; hydrocortisone 200 mg (IM or slow IV); nebulised salbutamol 2.5–5.0 mg; crystalloid 500–1000 ml IV.

Amniotic fluid embolism

Amniotic fluid embolism is a rare and largely unavoidable condition, and fortunately in the UK there has been a recent reduction in maternal deaths secondary to this condition. The incidence of maternal death in the last triennium was 0.57/100 000 maternities.[2] The condition occurs when amniotic fluid enters the maternal circulation, causing maternal collapse, and often leads to cardiac arrest. The woman is often conscious at the onset of symptoms. Presentation is acute with shivering, sweating, anxiety and coughing, followed by respiratory distress and cardiovascular collapse (hypotension, tachycardia and possible arrhythmias). DIC can quickly develop, causing massive maternal haemorrhage.

Diagnosis must initially be presumptive. Treatment involves support for the respiratory and cardiovascular systems and correction of clotting abnormalities. Early liaison with haematology staff is vital.

If the woman survives, diagnosis can be confirmed by identification of vernix, fetal hair or fetal squames from the maternal right-sided circulation. Fetal squames have been recovered in the maternal sputum in some cases. The presence of pulmonary hypertension may also be demonstrated.

Air embolism

An air embolism may occur following a ruptured uterus, during administration of intravenous fluids or blood products under pressure, or following manipulation of the placenta at caesarean section. Air embolism is associated with chest pain and collapse. An important differentiating factor from amniotic fluid embolism is the auscultation of a typical waterwheel murmur over the precordium.

References

1.   Lewis G (editor). The Confidential Enquiry into Maternal and Child Health (CEMACH). *Saving Mothers' Lives: Reviewing Maternal Deaths to Make Motherhood Safer 2003–2005. The Seventh Report on Confidential Enquiries into Maternal Deaths in the United Kingdom.* London: CEMACH; 2007.

2.   Centre for Maternal and Child Enquiries. Saving Mothers' Lives: reviewing maternal deaths to make motherhood safer: 2006–08. The Eighth Report on Confidential Enquiries into Maternal Deaths in the United Kingdom. *BJOG* 2011;118 Suppl 1:1–203.

3.   Resuscitation Council (UK) [www.resus.org.uk].

Module 3
Maternal cardiac arrest and advanced life support

Key learning points

- Management of cardiac arrest using advanced life support (ALS) algorithm.
- Recall the causes of maternal cardiac arrest.
- Keeping woman supine but using manual left uterine displacement to reduce aortocaval compression during CPR (or 30-degree left-lateral tilt if on a firm tilting surface, e.g. operating table).
- Perform perimortem caesarean or instrumental birth.
- Document details of management accurately, clearly and legibly.

Common difficulties observed in training drills

- Concentrating on ALS and forgetting to perform basic life support.
- Not tilting mother or manually displacing the uterus.
- Not connecting the defibrillator.
- Stopping cardiac compressions when new staff arrive or other actions are being performed.
- Lack of understanding that perimortem caesarean section is primarily performed for maternal resuscitation.
- Forgetting to call the neonatal team.

Introduction

Maternal cardiac arrest is rare and survival is low because of the physiological changes present in late pregnancy, which often hamper effective cardiopulmonary resuscitative efforts.

This module gives a brief outline of advanced life support but is not intended to be a complete guide to advanced resuscitation techniques. More information and specific training is available from the Resuscitation Council (UK)[1] and the European Resuscitation Council.[2]

The aim of this module is to provide maternity staff with an initial overview of advanced life support in relation to the pregnant woman.

Possible obstetric and anaesthetic causes of cardiac arrest during pregnancy and postpartum include:

- haemorrhage
- pre-eclampsia/eclampsia
- pulmonary embolism
- amniotic fluid embolism
- septicaemia
- total spinal anaesthesia
- local anaesthetic toxicity
- magnesium overdose.

These causes should be considered in addition to other causes of cardiac arrest in the non-pregnant woman (such as cardiac disease, substance abuse, anaphylaxis, trauma). Potentially reversible causes of cardiac arrest (the four Hs and the four Ts) are discussed later in this module.

Cardiorespiratory changes in pregnancy

In the supine position, pressure from the gravid uterus causes aortocaval compression. At term, the inferior vena cava is completely occluded in 90% of supine women, resulting in a decrease in cardiac stroke volume (the amount of blood pumped out with each contraction of the heart) of up to 70%. This has a significant effect on the cardiac output that can be achieved during cardiopulmonary resuscitation (CPR).

Therefore, to ensure that aortocaval compression is kept to a minimum while still maintaining good-quality, effective chest compressions, the woman should be kept supine with the uterus manually displaced to the left

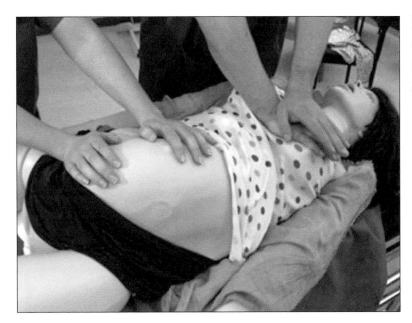

Figure 3.1 Manual displacement of the uterus to the left while administering CPR

by an assistant using one or two hands (Figure 3.1).[3] Alternatively, if the woman is on an operating table or another firm surface that can be tilted, e.g. a spinal board, then this can be tilted up to 30 degrees to the left.

If, by 5 minutes of effective CPR, resuscitation has not been successful, the baby's birth should be expedited. If the woman is fully dilated and the baby is easily deliverable vaginally, an instrumental birth should be performed; otherwise, a perimortem caesarean section should be undertaken. This will immediately relieve the vena caval obstruction caused by the gravid uterus and improves survival rates for both mother and infant.[4-6]

The pregnant woman at term has a 20% decrease in pulmonary functional residual capacity and a 20% increase in oxygen consumption. She therefore becomes hypoxic more rapidly than the non-pregnant woman.[7] The enlarged uterus, together with the resultant upward displacement of the abdominal organs, decreases lung compliance during ventilation, which makes adequate ventilation during cardiac arrest difficult.

Pregnancy increases the risk of pulmonary aspiration of gastric contents. Early tracheal intubation reduces this risk. However, oxygenation of the patient always takes priority and prolonged attempts at intubation should be avoided.

Management of maternal cardiac arrest

An algorithm for the management of maternal cardiac arrest is shown in Figure 3.2. A fuller list of the actions required in the event of maternal cardiac arrest is given in Box 3.1 (page 30).

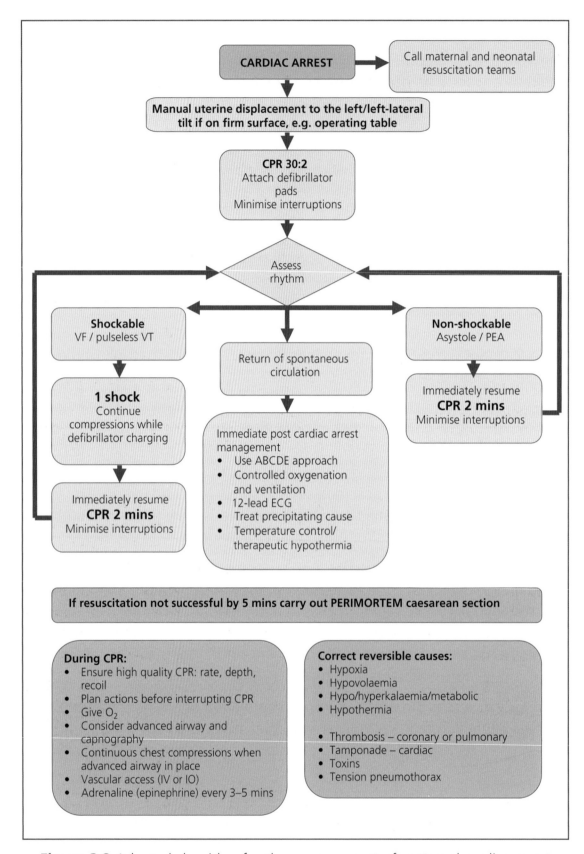

Figure 3.2 Adapted algorithm for the management of maternal cardiac arrest

Role of the team leader

The team leader is usually a doctor on the cardiac arrest team; however, it could be anybody trained in advanced life support. The team leader should direct the team and ensure their safety. This is best achieved by standing back, delegating specific tasks to members of the team and ensuring that clear commands are given. The team leader must consider any correctable cause of cardiac arrest and decide whether administering any other drugs (Table 3.1) may be beneficial.

Table 3.1 Drugs to be considered during cardiac arrest

Feature	Drug to be considered
Cardiac arrest	1 mg adrenaline (epinephrine) IV every 3–5 minutes
VF/VT	300 mg amiodarone IV after third shock
Opiate overdose	0.4–0.8 mg naloxone IV
Magnesium toxicity	1 g calcium gluconate (10 ml of 10% solution) IV
Bupivacaine toxicity	1.5 ml/kg intralipid 20% IV initially

Drugs should be administered via the intravenous or intraosseous route. The tracheal route is no longer recommended.

In a maternal cardiac arrest, it is important for the team leader (or any other members of the team) to state immediately after arrest occurs that a perimortem delivery (by caesarean section unless the woman is fully dilated) will need to be performed within 5 minutes of commencing CPR, if resuscitation has not been successful. The equipment required to assist birth should be immediately prepared (Figure 3.3; page 32). The neonatal team will be required to resuscitate the baby and, hence, it is important to call them as soon as a maternal arrest occurs so they have time to prepare equipment.

> **It is important to continue with CPR throughout the caesarean section or instrumental birth.**

The cardiac arrest team leader should decide when a resuscitation attempt should be abandoned. This should be done in consultation with the rest of the team. The team leader is also responsible for documenting the arrest and ensuring that staff and relatives are well supported afterwards.

It is good practice to ensure someone remains with the relatives during an arrest and keeps them as informed as possible.

Box 3.1 Management of maternal cardiac arrest	
EVENT	**ACTION**
Help	■ Shout for help ■ **Ring 2222** and state '**maternal cardiac arrest**' and location of the incident ■ Ask for the arrest trolley, perimortem caesarean section pack and resuscitaire ■ **Call neonatal team (if pregnant woman)** ■ Ensure security doors are open so that arrest team can arrive ■ Contact blood bank and ask for emergency blood products ■ Phone haematology and biochemistry for urgent blood test requests
Positioning	■ Lay the bed flat ■ Ask assistant to manually displace the uterus to the left (or tilt woman 30 degrees to the left if on a firm tilting surface, e.g. operating table). ■ Move the bed into the centre of the room ■ Take head end off the bed
Basic life support	■ Open airway ■ Give 30 chest compressions (at rate of 100–120 compressions/minute) in middle of lower half of sternum to a depth of 5–6 cm: the emphasis is on good-quality chest compressions with regard to rate, depth and recoil ■ Next, give 2 breaths using a pocket mask or bag/mask ventilation ■ Continue at ratio of 30 chest compressions to 2 breaths (each breath lasting 1 second)
Equipment	■ **Defibrillator** – immediately apply gel pads and view rhythm to decide if a shock should be given: continue chest compressions while pads are applied ■ Deliver shock if appropriate; CONTINUE chest compressions while defibrillator is charging or, if using an AED, follow instructions ■ **Perimortem delivery equipment** – open perimortem caesarean pack and disposable scalpel or instrumental set, and be ready to deliver baby at 5 minutes if CPR unsuccessful; alert theatre team ■ **Resuscitaire** must be turned on

Box 3.1 Management of maternal cardiac arrest (continued)

EVENT	ACTION
Investigations	■ **Large-bore IV access** should be obtained as soon as possible ■ **Venous blood** – send urgently for FBC, U&Es, LFTs, clotting screen, cross-matching, calcium and magnesium ■ **Arterial blood gas** – some units may have blood gas analysers which will give immediate estimates of haemoglobin, K^+, Na^+, Ca^{2+} and glucose as well as pH, PaO_2 and $PaCO_2$
Advanced life support	■ As soon as the arrest team arrives, a team leader should be appointed. In most hospitals a predetermined member of the arrest team assumes this role. They should coordinate the arrest including allocating specific tasks to members of the team ■ CPR should be uninterrupted, except for shocks and rhythm checks (where appropriate), including during caesarean section, if required ■ The anaesthetist will normally manage the airway/breathing. Once the woman is intubated, chest compressions should be continuous. Capnography should be considered. ■ **Shocks** – every 2 minutes if VF/pulseless VT ■ **Adrenaline (epinephrine)** – 1 mg IV flushed with at least 20 ml of 0.9% saline or water for injections (depending on local maternal resuscitation guidelines) (after 3rd shock if VF/pulseless VT), repeated every 3–5 minutes
Deliver the baby	■ If resuscitation has not been successful by 5 minutes, deliver by quickest means (caesarean section or forceps) ■ Continue CPR during operation ■ Ensure the neonatal team is in attendance
Documentation	■ Note the time of the arrest, arrival of staff, timing of defibrillation, timing of drugs administered, time of delivery of baby and time cardiac output is regained

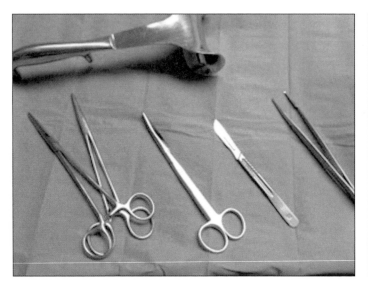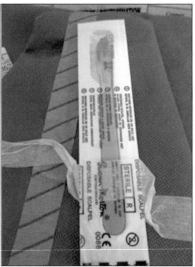

Figure 3.3 Equipment required for perimortem caesarean section, with disposable scalpel attached to outside of pack

Recognition of heart rhythms

Resuscitation attempts should follow the predetermined evidence-based algorithms published by the Resuscitation Council (UK).[1] The advanced life support algorithm (Figure 3.2; page 28) has two main pathways: those requiring direct current cardioversion ('shockable rhythms') and those in which this would be inappropriate ('non-shockable rhythms') (Box 3.2). The cardiac rhythm dictates which pathway to follow.

Box 3.2 Heart rhythms found during cardiac arrest	
Shockable rhythms	**Non-shockable rhythms**
Ventricular fibrillation (VF)	Asystole
Pulseless ventricular tachycardia (VT)	Pulseless electrical activity (PEA)

Once cardiac arrest is confirmed, a defibrillator should be used to rapidly assess the cardiac rhythm of the woman. Self-adhesive pads are placed on the woman's chest and may be used for both cardiac monitoring and/or defibrillation. Do not stop chest compressions to apply the pads.

The ECG leads are colour coded and should be attached with the red electrode to the right shoulder (Red to Right), the yellow electrode to the left shoulder (yeLLow to Left) and the green electrode below the pectoral muscles (green for spleen) (Figure 3.4). The defibrillator should be altered to read the ECG rhythm through lead two. Alternatively, the cardiac rhythm may be viewed through the self-adhesive defibrillator pads attached to the woman's chest, as illustrated in Figure 3.4.

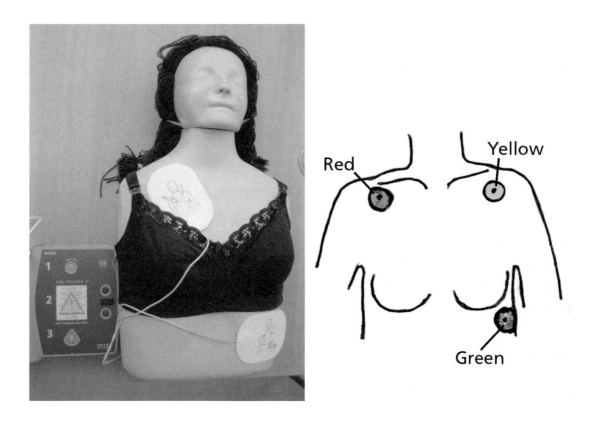

Figure 3.4 Defibrillation pads and ECG electrode placement

During arrest, the heart rhythms seen will fit into one of the two categories: shockable or non-shockable (Box 3.2; page 32).

Shockable rhythms

The majority of survivors from cardiac arrests come from the shockable rhythm category (VF and pulseless VT). A typical example of VF is shown in Figure 3.5.

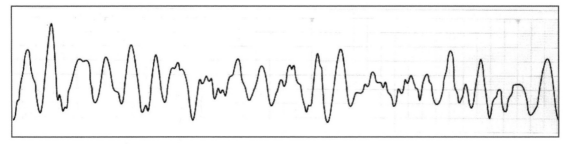

Figure 3.5 An example of ventricular fibrillation

VT is characterised by a broad-complex regular tachycardia (Figure 3.6). VT can cause a profound loss of cardiac output and can suddenly deteriorate into VF. Pulseless VT is treated in the same way as VF.

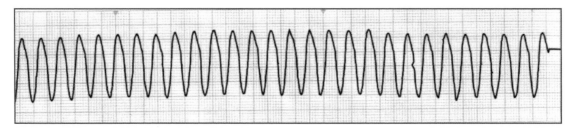

Figure 3.6 Ventricular tachycardia

Shockable cardiac rhythms need to be treated by defibrillation. This involves passing an electrical current across the heart to simultaneously depolarise a critical mass of the myocardium so that the natural pacemaking tissue of the heart can resume control. Attempted defibrillation is the single most important step in the treatment of VF/VT. The time between the onset of VF/VT and defibrillation is the main determinant of patient survival. Survival falls by 7–10% for each minute following collapse.

Most defibrillators now transmit a biphasic current, which has a higher efficiency, so less energy is required to depolarise the heart. When using a biphasic defibrillator, a current of 150–200 Joules (J) should be used for the first shock, and 150–360 J for subsequent shocks; for a monophasic defibrillator, 360 J should be used for the first and subsequent shocks.

Know your machine: if unsure, shock at 200 J.

Remember: only one shock per cycle is given for shockable rhythms; the shock is then immediately followed by 2 minutes of CPR at a ratio of 30 compressions to 2 ventilations (without checking for a rhythm or a pulse). After 2 minutes, the rhythm should be checked and a second shock delivered, if required. A pulse should be checked only if a non-shockable rhythm is seen.

> **Adrenaline (epinephrine) 1 mg IV should be given after alternate shocks (every 3–5 minutes, starting immediately after the third shock).**
>
> **Amiodarone 300 mg IV should also be given after the third shock.**

Most clinical areas now have automated external defibrillators (AEDs), which are able to analyse the cardiac rhythm and deliver appropriate shocks if indicated.

It is important to continue chest compressions while the defibillator is charging, prior to the delivery of the shock. If using an AED, follow the machine's instructions. Figure 3.7 shows an example of an AED used for training.

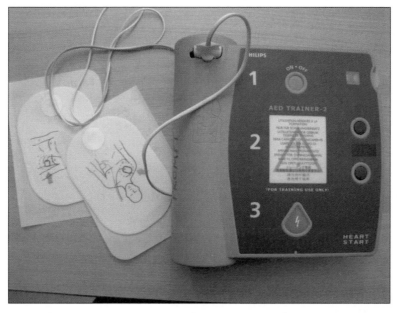

Figure 3.7 An example of an AED machine used for training

Non-shockable rhythms

Pulseless electrical activity (PEA) signifies the clinical absence of cardiac output (i.e. no pulse) despite cardiac electrical activity, which may be normal (sinus rhythm or near normal). For example, in exsanguination, the heart's electrical activity may continue to show a normal sinus rhythm, as shown in Figure 3.8, but there is no circulating blood so a pulse is not present.

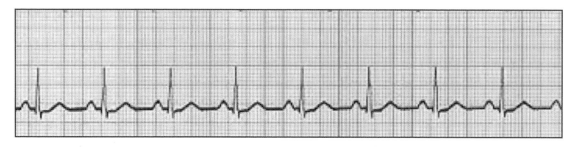

Figure 3.8 Normal sinus rhythm or electrical activity which can be found in pulseless electrical activity

Asystole is a slightly wandering flat line; an example is shown in Figure 3.9. Until proven otherwise a completely flat horizontal line indicates that the monitoring leads are not correctly attached rather than asystole. Adults in asystole have a very poor prognosis.

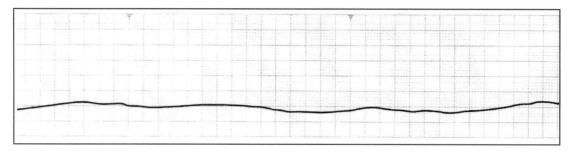

Figure 3.9 Asystole

- **If there is any doubt about whether the rhythm is asystole or fine VF, do not attempt defibrillation; instead, continue chest compressions and ventilation 30:2.**
- **Adrenaline (epinephrine) 1 mg IV should be given as soon as possible and then every 3–5 minutes.**

Potentially reversible causes

If the cardiac rhythm is not VF or VT, the outcome will be poor unless a potentially reversible cause can be found and treated. Potentially reversible causes of cardiac arrest can be remembered using the four 'Hs' and four 'Ts'.

The four Hs

1. **Hypoxia** should be minimised by ensuring that the patient is adequately ventilated during the arrest. Basic life support followed by prompt intubation and ventilation using 100% oxygen should maximise oxygen delivery to the woman. She should be examined to check for chest rise and bilateral air entry during ventilation.

2. **Hypovolaemia** is most commonly caused by massive haemorrhage (such as abruption or postpartum haemorrhage). Intravenous fluids and blood products should be started promptly to restore the intravascular volume and urgent surgery to correct the cause of bleeding should be considered.

3. **Hypo/hyperkalaemia/metabolic**

    ■ **Hypoglycaemia** may occur in a diabetic mother. If the blood glucose measures below 3 mmol/l, give 50 ml of 20% glucose solution IV.

    ■ **Hyperkalaemia** (high serum potassium) can develop secondary to renal failure.

    ■ **Hypermagnesaemia** (high serum magnesium) may result from treatment of pre-eclampsia with intravenous magnesium sulphate, especially with concurrent renal impairment.

    ■ **Hypocalcaemia** (low serum calcium) can result from overdose of calcium channel blocking drugs such as nifedipine.

    High serum levels of potassium or magnesium and low serum levels of calcium should be treated with 10 ml of 10% calcium gluconate IV.

4. **Hypothermia** is an unlikely cause of maternal arrest in hospital. Attempts should be made to keep patients warm in the peri-arrest situation by using warmed intravenous fluids and warming blankets if appropriate. However, once cardiac arrest has occurred, mild therapeutic hypothermia (to 35 degrees) can provide neuroprotection.[8]

The four Ts

1. **Thromboemboli** are more common in pregnancy owing to the procoagulant effect of pregnancy and the mechanical obstruction to venous return caused by the gravid uterus. Massive pulmonary embolus can cause sudden collapse and cardiac arrest. Treatment is difficult but thrombolysis, cardiopulmonary bypass or operative removal of the clot should be considered. Amniotic fluid emboli are also a cause of sudden collapse and cardiac arrest. Treatment remains supportive and care should be taken to correct clotting abnormalities as disseminated

intravascular coagulopathy often results. Early liaison with haematology is essential.

2. **Tension pneumothorax** can cause collapse and subsequent PEA. A tension pneumothorax is most likely to occur during attempted central venous line insertion or trauma. Treatment involves acute decompression of the affected side by inserting a large intravenous cannula into the thoracic cavity in the second intercostal space at the midclavicular line, followed by chest drain insertion.

3. **Therapeutic** or **toxic** substances (for example, inadvertent administration of bupivacaine intravenously or opiate overdose) can cause arrest. Specific antidotes or treatments should be used; for example, for opiate overdose, naloxone 0.4–0.8 mg IV or, for bupivacaine overdose, IV intralipid.

4. Cardiac **tamponade** is an uncommon cause of maternal arrest but should be considered in trauma, especially when there are penetrating chest injuries. Treatment involves relieving the tamponade by needle pericardiocentesis.

Drugs used during cardiac arrest

Adrenaline (epinephrine) 1 mg should be given IV every 3–5 minutes during a cardiac arrest. Other drugs that may be considered are listed in Table 3.1; page 29.

All drugs should be flushed with at least 20ml of 0.9% saline or water for injections (depending on local maternal resuscitation guidelines) to ensure they enter the central circulation. The most common drugs required for a cardiac arrest are kept on the resuscitation trolley in prefilled syringes, so that they can be quickly administered in an emergency. It is important that all staff are aware of the location of the emergency trolley and defibrillator within their own unit. It is also important that staff familiarise themselves with the use of their local emergency equipment and drugs, as equipment may vary between locations.

Post-resuscitation care

A comprehensive, structured post-resuscitation protocol is important and would normally include transfer to an intensive care unit:

■ ABCDE approach.
■ Controlled oxygenation and ventilation. Consideration should be given to avoiding hyperoxia. Inspired oxygen should be titrated to maintain

- Temperature and glucose control. Consideration should be given to the use of therapeutic hypothermia. Glucose levels greater than 10 mmol/l should be treated but hypoglycemia avoided.
- A 12-lead ECG should be performed.
- Precipitating causes should be treated.

References

1. Resuscitation Council (UK) [www.resus.org.uk].
2. European Resuscitation Council [www.erc.edu].
3. Resuscitation Council (UK). FAQs on advanced life support. 2012 [www.resus.org.uk/page/faqALS.htm].
4. Marx G. Cardiopulmonary resuscitation of late-pregnant women. *Anaesthesiology* 1982;56:156.
5. Oates S, Williams GL, Res GA. Cardiopulmonary resuscitation in late pregnancy. *Br Med J* 1988;297:404–5.
6. Page-Rodriguez A, Gonzalez-Sanchez JA. Perimortem caesarean section of twin pregnancy: case report and review of the literature. *Acad Emerg Med* 1999;6:1072–4.
7. Zakowski MI, Ramanathan S. CPR in pregnancy. *Curr Rev Clin Anesth* 1990;10:106.
8. Arrich J, Holzer M, Herkner H, Müllner M. Hypothermia for neuroprotection in adults after cardiopulmonary resuscitation. *Cochrane Database Syst Rev* 2009;(4):CD004128.

Module 4
Maternal anaesthetic emergencies

Key learning points

- To understand the difficulties of intubation in the obstetric patient.
- To understand the management of failed intubation.
- Recognition and management of high regional block.
- Signs and symptoms of local anaesthetic toxicity.
- Management of cardiac arrest in a patient with local anaesthetic toxicity.

Background

In the Confidential Enquiry into Maternal Deaths in the United Kingdom 2006–08, 50% of the women who died from either direct or indirect causes had been given an anaesthetic. Of the 127 deaths attributable to direct causes, seven (3%) were attributed to anaesthesia.[1] This is a slightly increased mortality rate over that seen in the previous triennium (0.31/100 000 maternities). It is disappointing to note that in all six cases in the 2006–08 triennium, it was thought that care was substandard. There were a further 18 direct and indirect deaths in which perioperative or anaesthesia management contributed, and a further 12 cases of severe pregnancy-induced hypertension or sepsis where obstetricians or gynaecologists failed to consult with anaesthetic or critical care services sufficiently early.[1]

The role of the anaesthetist in the multidisciplinary team involves unique challenges: their specific skills are often required in high-stress situations when time is critical and maternal or fetal life is at risk. It is in these circumstances that help from the rest of the maternity team can be invaluable.

Failed tracheal intubation

Introduction

General anaesthesia for caesarean section is now uncommon. Of the 157 359 caesarean sections carried out in England and Wales during 2009 and 2010, less than 5% (7531) were performed under general anaesthetic. The vast majority of general anaesthetics were performed in emergency cases (6209; 84.4%).[2] Box 4.1 outlines the indications for general anaesthesia.

Box 4.1 Indications for general anaesthesia

- Severe maternal or fetal compromise requiring immediate delivery
- Regional anaesthesia contraindicated (e.g. coagulopathy, haemodynamic instability)
- Failed regional anaesthesia
- Maternal request

The majority of complications arising from general anaesthesia relate to the airway. When the airway needs to be secured in an obstetric patient, it is important that endotracheal intubation (a tube with a cuff placed through, and secured below, the vocal cords to maintain a patent airway) is used, as pregnant women are at increased risk of regurgitation and aspiration of gastric contents.

A failed intubation is an anaesthetic emergency and can be defined in a number of ways. A useful definition for the maternity team is: a failed intubation has occurred when the anaesthetist has been unable to insert the endotracheal tube after two attempts. It is at this point that the failed intubation drill will begin and help will be required from the rest of the team, although it would be prudent to prepare to assist the anaesthetist after the first failed attempt at intubation.

Failed intubation is more common in the obstetric population than in the general surgical population (1 in 250 in pregnancy compared with 1 in 2200 in general surgical patients). This is because intubation is more difficult in pregnancy for several reasons, including complete dentition (i.e. most pregnant women have a full set of teeth), increased pharyngeal and laryngeal oedema, the larger tongue of pregnancy and the larger breasts associated with pregnancy. In addition, pregnant women rapidly desaturate owing to the additional oxygen requirements of pregnancy.[3] The rising level of obesity is likely to make intubation of pregnant women even more difficult in the future.

Ideally, all difficult intubations would be predicted antenatally so that a plan could be made before the event. An antenatal assessment should aim to identify women who may be at risk of a difficult intubation and referral to an obstetric anaesthetist should be arranged (Box 4.2).

Box 4.2 Risk factors for difficult intubation

- Known previous difficult intubation
- Obesity
- Pre-eclampsia
- Congenital airway difficulties with restricted neck movement and limited mouth opening (e.g. Klippel–Feil syndrome, Pierre Robin syndrome)
- Acquired airway difficulties with restricted neck movement and limited mouth opening (e.g. rheumatoid arthritis, ankylosing spondylitis, cervical spine fusions)

Unfortunately, most tests used to identify patients with potentially difficult airways are unreliable, particularly in the obstetric population. As a result, anaesthetists may be faced with an unexpectedly difficult or impossible intubation. To minimise complications during these infrequent events, it helps to use a clear algorithm.

Management and reduction of potential complications

The management of failed intubation in the obstetric patient should involve early recognition of the potentially difficult airway. For example, some recommend inserting an epidural early in labour for morbidly obese mothers.[4] This provides the option of an epidural top-up should an emergency caesarean section be required, as a rapid spinal at this stage would be technically difficult and more likely to fail.

Aspiration of gastric contents is more likely during difficult intubation, in emergency cases and in obese pregnant patients. For this reason, particular attention should be paid to reducing the volume and acidity of stomach contents in high-risk women during labour. Local guidelines should be in place for high-risk women (e.g. in cases of obesity) which recommend limiting food intake during labour. Isotonic sports drinks may be encouraged and regular prophylactic H_2 receptor antagonists given (e.g. oral ranitidine 150 mg 6-hourly). These prophylactic measures provide another safeguard to reduce the potential morbidity and mortality associated with emergency obstetric surgery and anaesthesia.

In the event of an emergency general anaesthetic, preparation can make the difference between success and failure at intubation. Optimal positioning of the mother is paramount, particularly in the morbidly obese woman. The mother's head should be as near to the anaesthetist as possible, with pillows positioned so that the mother's neck is flexed and her chin is pointing up towards the ceiling (Figure 4.1).

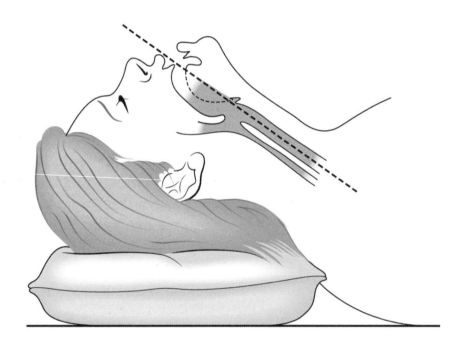

Figure 4.1 Optimal anatomical position for successful laryngoscopy

In pregnant women, and in particular those with large breasts or who are obese, it can be useful to adopt the 'ramped' position. This has been shown to improve the view of the vocal cords at laryngoscopy, making intubation easier.[5] The ramped position aims to create a horizontal line between the sternal notch and the external auditory meatus, as shown in Figure 4.2. The position can be achieved using purpose-made pillows such as the Oxford HELP (Head Elevating Laryngoscopy Pillow) or by adjusting the operating table and using extra pillows and wedges.

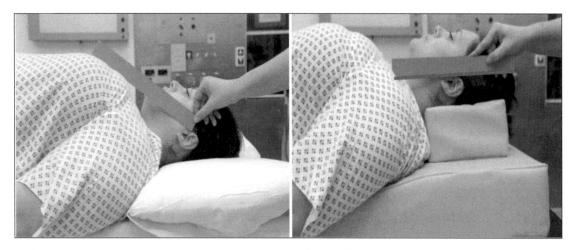

Figure 4.2 Anatomical realignment using the Oxford HELP to improve intubating conditions (© Alma Medical Products 2010, reproduced with permission)

Once the woman is positioned on the operating table, pre-oxygenation will begin. Pre-oxygenation is important to prevent desaturation during intubation, which can occur rapidly in pregnant women. The aim is to fill the lungs with as much oxygen as possible and remove nitrogen so that, when the patient is rendered apnoeic (i.e. has stopped breathing) upon induction of anaesthesia, there is enough oxygen available for gaseous exchange for the period of time it takes to secure the endotracheal tube and commence mechanical ventilation. For effective pre-oxygenation, the face mask must be tightly applied to the patient's face, not leaving any room for air to enter and dilute the oxygen delivered. At this stage, help from the team to attach monitoring equipment, cannulate the patient and prepare the abdomen and drapes can maximise time for pre-oxygenation while minimising time to delivery.

It is important for members of the theatre team to remain quiet during induction of anaesthesia, and to be prepared to help in the event of a failed intubation. If failed intubation has occurred, the anaesthetist should immediately declare the emergency and state 'this is a failed intubation'. Individual roles will vary during the emergency. The anaesthetist and operating department practitioner will be unable to leave the woman, so other team members will be needed to provide assistance. All staff in theatre should know where the difficult airway equipment is kept and be able to fetch it if requested. All staff in theatre should also know how to call for additional anaesthetic support. A failed intubation is inevitably a very stressful situation in which clear communication will be essential.

The failed intubation algorithm is outlined in Figure 4.3 (page 47).

In the event of a failed intubation, the life of the woman is the anaesthetist's priority. In most cases the woman must be woken up, but in exceptional circumstances it might be considered appropriate to continue with surgery if oxygenation and ventilation are possible.

Under these circumstances, the procedure will be performed under general anaesthesia but the patient may well be spontaneously breathing without muscle relaxation. The caesarean section will therefore be technically more difficult, as gaining access to the uterus can be problematic and the use of high concentrations of anaesthetic gases may cause uterine relaxation, thus increasing the risk of haemorrhage. The most senior obstetrician should perform the surgery as quickly as possible to limit the anaesthetic time.

Box 4.3 outlines best practice points for tracheal intubation.

Box 4.3 Best practice points for tracheal intubation

- Identify women at risk and refer for antenatal anaesthetic assessment
- Assess the airway before induction of anaesthesia
- Anaesthetists and operating department practitioners should check all intubation and difficult airway equipment daily and be familiar with its use and location
- Position the patient correctly before induction
- Pre-oxygenate carefully
- Call for help early
- Remember that oxygenation is more important than intubation

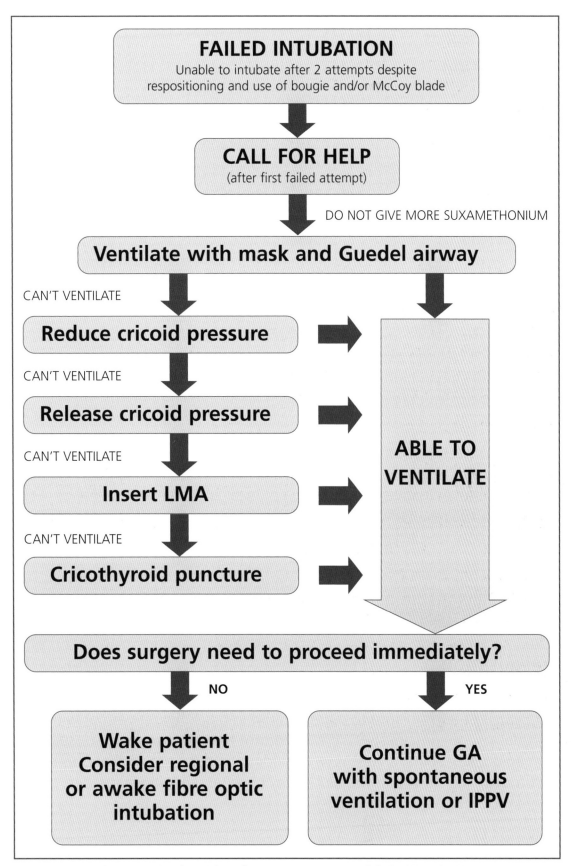

Figure 4.3 Algorithm for management of failed intubation
(adapted from North Bristol NHS Trust Guideline 2004)

High regional block

Introduction

An excessively high block following spinal or epidural anaesthesia that requires the patient to be intubated has been described as 'the failed intubation of the new millennium'.[6] This is because, as the use of general anaesthesia has decreased, the use of regional anaesthesia has increased, thus increasing the incidence of high regional block.

The height of the block following spinal or epidural anaesthesia varies between patients. The term 'high block' encompasses a spectrum of clinical events. At one end of the spectrum a patient may exhibit mild symptoms and only require reassurance with or without supplemental oxygen; at the other end, the patient may stop breathing, which may lead to cardiac arrest.

The term 'total spinal' implies that unconsciousness has also occurred. Total spinal is defined as cardiorespiratory collapse caused by direct action of local anaesthetic on high cervical nerve roots and the brainstem. It is a rare complication of epidural anaesthesia with an incidence of approximately 1 in 16 000.[7,8]

A high regional block can inadvertently occur in a number of ways. It can be an exaggerated response to correctly placed and dosed local anaesthetic, or attributable to an inadvertent overdose of local anaesthetic at spinal or epidural, or the result of accidental injection of local anaesthetic into the wrong space (e.g. subdural or intrathecal injection of an epidural dose).

> **A total spinal or a high block with inadequate breathing requiring intubation are both anaesthetic emergencies.**

Presentation

The presentation of high regional block can vary from rapid loss of consciousness and collapse to a gradual rise in block height with or without eventual loss of consciousness. It is important to monitor women closely after epidural or spinal anaesthesia (including epidural top-ups) and to be alert to warning signs that the block may be extending above the desired height (Box 4.4).

Box 4.4 Warning signs of rising block

- Nausea
- 'Not feeling right'
- Breathlessness
- Tingling fingers or arms
- Difficulty speaking
- Difficulty swallowing
- Sedation

Some women will have a block that reaches the lower cervical nerve roots, especially after spinal anaesthesia. Reassurance is often all that is necessary, but it is important to call for help, observe the woman closely, assess her pulse, blood pressure, respiratory rate and oxygen saturations and look for the warning signs outlined in Box 4.4.

If the local anaesthetic reaches the upper cervical nerve roots and blocks the nerves supplying the diaphragm, the woman will have great difficulty breathing and rapidly become hypoxic. In addition, if the brainstem is affected (total spinal), there is also likely to be severe hypotension and bradycardia. Fetal bradycardia may occur as a result of reduced placental blood flow.

There are several risk factors for high regional block, which mean it is not a complication confined to the theatre environment where an anaesthetist would be present (Box 4.5). High regional block should be in the differential diagnosis for maternal collapse in any woman receiving an epidural.

Box 4.5 Risk factors for high regional block

- Accidental dural puncture (recognised or unrecognised) during epidural insertion
- Accidental subdural placement of epidural catheter
- Large or rapid epidural top-ups (e.g. for category 1 caesarean section)
- Spinal injection with epidural in place
- Epidural top-ups after recent spinal injection

Management

In the situation where a woman exhibits warning signs of a high block (Box 4.4), it is imperative to remain with her and to call for help early in case she continues to deteriorate (Figure 4.4).

In the event of a high block with inadequate ventilation or a total spinal, characterised by cardiorespiratory collapse, the emergency buzzer should be used to summon help immediately. It may be necessary to call the maternal cardiac arrest team to ensure that enough skilled people are present to

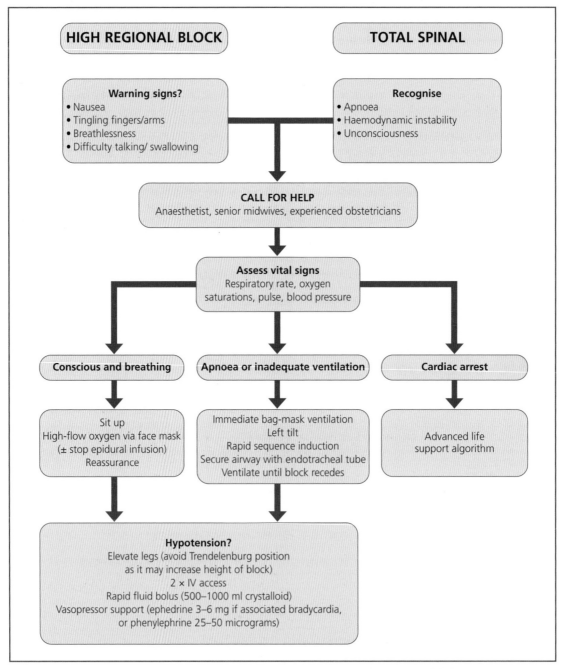

Figure 4.4 Management algorithm for high regional block

intubate the patient, manage ventilation and provide circulatory support, deliver the baby and give advanced life support if cardiac arrest ensues (see **Module 2** and **Module 3**).

Remember: call for help, assess ABC and deliver 100% oxygen.

The woman should be intubated and ventilated. Circulatory support, in the form of intravenous fluids, vasopressors and inotropes, will be necessary, particularly if there is a total spinal. The hypotension and bradycardia may be catastrophic and can result in cardiac arrest, in which case chest compressions should be commenced immediately (with manual left uterine displacement or left-lateral tilt) and advanced life support instituted. Following a total spinal, even without cardiac arrest, the baby is likely to be compromised as a result of maternal hypoxia and hypotension, and this may necessitate urgent delivery.

Once the woman has been resuscitated, anaesthetic agents will be needed to keep her asleep as she may be conscious but, owing to the paralysing effect of the block, unable to move or communicate. The effect of the block may last for less than 1 hour or may take several hours to wear off. It may be possible to manage this situation in the operating theatre, or the woman may require transfer to the intensive care unit.

Local anaesthetic toxicity

Introduction

Local anaesthetics are widely used in obstetric anaesthetic practice. During 2009–10 there were over 180 000 spinal or epidural anaesthetics performed in England and Wales alone.[2] As with all interventions, local anaesthetics are not without risk and have been associated with deaths. One of the six deaths attributable to anaesthesia reported in the Confidential Enquiry into Maternal Deaths 2003–05 was the result of a drug administration error:[1]

> 'A woman of slight build had a low dose infusion epidural during labour and was delivered by forceps. She had some bleeding and intravenous fluid and syntocinon infusions were started. Shortly after she had a grand mal convulsion followed by ventricular fibrillation from which she could not be resuscitated. She had received 150 ml of a 500 ml bag of 0.1% bupivacaine in saline intravenously in error.'

This was a system error as a bag of epidural bupivacaine should never have been confused with a bag of intravenous fluid. Nevertheless, this tragic case demonstrates the danger of local anaesthetics if administered intravascularly.

The National Reporting and Learning Service of the National Patient Safety Agency (NPSA) has since published several safety alerts advising on strategies to avoid such errors. Initial recommendations focused on clear labelling and the use of equipment specifically designed for epidural injections and infusions.[9] Further recommendations stated that by 1 April 2012 all spinal (intrathecal) injections needed to be performed using syringes, needles and other devices with connectors that would not also connect with intravenous equipment.[10] This will be extended to all epidural and regional anaesthesia infusions and bolus doses by 1 April 2013.[11]

Signs and symptoms of local anaesthetic toxicity

Local anaesthetic toxicity can present in many different ways, making recognition difficult. It is particularly important to remember that, after a bolus dose, toxicity may occur at any point within the next hour. In units where epidural infusions are used during labour, toxicity could happen at any time. The features to look for are shown in Table 4.1.

Table 4.1 Signs and symptoms of toxicity

Warning signs	■ Tingling (mouth/tongue)	
	■ Metallic taste in the mouth	
	■ Ringing in the ears	
	■ Lightheadedness	
	■ Agitation ('just not right')	
	■ Tremor	
Severe toxicity	**Neurological**	**Cardiovascular**
	■ Severe agitation	■ Bradycardia
	■ Loss of consciousness	■ Heart block
	■ Convulsions	■ Ventricular tachyarrhythmias
		■ Asystole/cardiac arrest

Remember: the first sign may be cardiac arrest.

Management

All healthcare professionals caring for women with epidurals should be familiar with the management of severe local anaesthetic toxicity.[9] The Association of Anaesthetists of Great Britain and Ireland published guidelines in 2010, an outline of which is illustrated in Table 4.2. The lipid emulsion regimen is shown in Figure 4.5 (page 54). Further information can be found at www.aagbi.org and www.lipidrescue.org.

Table 4.2 Management of severe local anaesthetic toxicity

Immediate management	■ Stop injecting local anaesthetic ■ Call for help ■ Maintain airway; intubate if necessary ■ Give 100% oxygen and ensure adequate ventilation ■ Confirm/establish IV access ■ Control seizures ■ Assess cardiovascular status throughout

Treatment	**In cardiac arrest**
	■ Commence advanced life support using standard algorithm with woman supine and uterus manually displaced to the left
	■ Treat arrhythmias using standard protocols
	■ Give intravenous lipid emulsion (follow regimen shown in Figure 4.5)
	■ Continue CPR throughout treatment with lipid emulsion
	■ Recovery may take longer than 1 hour
	
	Without cardiac arrest
	■ Use conventional therapies to treat:
	  □ Hypotension
	  □ Bradycardia
	  □ Tachyarrhythmias
	■ Consider intravenous lipid emulsion
	■ Keep woman in left-lateral tilt

Special points	■ Propofol is not a suitable substitute for lipid emulsion ■ Arrhythmias may be very refractory to treatment ■ Lidocaine should not be used as an antiarrhythmic in this setting

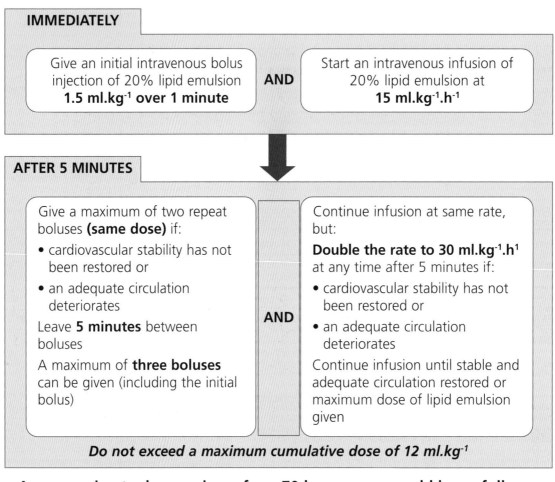

IMMEDIATELY

Give an initial intravenous bolus injection of 20% lipid emulsion **1.5 ml.kg⁻¹ over 1 minute**

AND

Start an intravenous infusion of 20% lipid emulsion at **15 ml.kg⁻¹.h⁻¹**

AFTER 5 MINUTES

Give a maximum of two repeat boluses **(same dose)** if:

• cardiovascular stability has not been restored or

• an adequate circulation deteriorates

Leave **5 minutes** between boluses

A maximum of **three boluses** can be given (including the initial bolus)

AND

Continue infusion at same rate, but:

Double the rate to 30 ml.kg⁻¹.h¹ at any time after 5 minutes if:

• cardiovascular stability has not been restored or

• an adequate circulation deteriorates

Continue infusion until stable and adequate circulation restored or maximum dose of lipid emulsion given

Do not exceed a maximum cumulative dose of 12 ml.kg⁻¹

An approximate dose regimen for a 70 kg woman would be as follows:

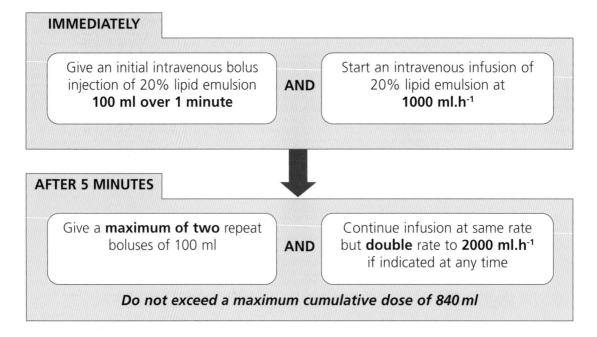

IMMEDIATELY

Give an initial intravenous bolus injection of 20% lipid emulsion **100 ml over 1 minute**

AND

Start an intravenous infusion of 20% lipid emulsion at **1000 ml.h⁻¹**

AFTER 5 MINUTES

Give a **maximum of two** repeat boluses of 100 ml

AND

Continue infusion at same rate but **double** rate to **2000 ml.h⁻¹** if indicated at any time

Do not exceed a maximum cumulative dose of 840 ml

Figure 4.5 Intravenous lipid emulsion regimen (© The Association of Anaesthetists of Great Britain & Ireland 2010, reproduced with permission)

Specific treatment for local anaesthetic toxicity

Local anaesthetic toxicity has successfully been treated with an intravenous infusion of lipid emulsion, commercially known as Intralipid® (Baxter Healthcare Corporation, Deerfield, IL, USA) in the UK. Intralipid has been reported to improve survival from local-anaesthetic-induced cardiac arrest[12,13] and in the treatment of life-threatening toxicity without cardiac arrest.[14] It does not replace the need for CPR, which should continue throughout treatment with lipid emulsion until the return of spontaneous circulation. It should be noted that cardiac arrest secondary to local anaesthetic toxicity can be refractory to treatment and recovery may take over 1 hour. Thus, the effort of a large number of people is required to ensure that good quality CPR is maintained throughout.

> **Remember: Know where lipid emulsion is kept in your department.**

Severe local anaesthetic toxicity is a rare but very serious complication of local anaesthetic use. Posters can be used in departments to remind staff of the salient points and, most importantly, where to find treatment guidelines and lipid emulsion should they ever be faced with this emergency.

Follow-up

The management of local-anaesthetic-induced cardiac arrest is very demanding. If successful, transfer to a critical care area will need to be arranged until full recovery is achieved.

Each case should be reported. The lessons learned can potentially prevent other cases from happening and improve our knowledge and treatment of the condition. In the UK, all cases should be reported to the NPSA, and cases where lipid has been given should be reported to the international registry at www.lipidregistry.org.

References

1. Centre for Maternal and Child Enquiries. Saving Mothers' Lives: reviewing maternal deaths to make motherhood safer: 2006–08. The Eighth Report on Confidential Enquiries into Maternal Deaths in the United Kingdom. *BJOG* 2011;118 Suppl 1:1–203.

2. Hospital Episode Statistics. NHS Maternity Statistics, 2009–2010. London: The Health and Social Care Information Centre; 2010 [http://www.hesonline.nhs.uk/Ease/servlet/ContentServer?siteID=1937&categoryID=1804].

3. McGlennan A, Mustafa A. General anaesthesia for Caesarean section. *Contin Educ Anaesth Crit Care Pain* 2009;9:148–51.

4. Centre for Maternal and Child Enquiries, Royal College of Obstetricians and Gynaecologists. *CMACE/RCOG Joint Guideline. Management of Women with Obesity in Pregnancy*. London: CMACE/RCOG; 2010 [http://www.rcog.org.uk/womens-health/clinical-guidance/management-women-obesity-pregnancy].

5. Collins JS, Lemmens HJ, Brodsky JB, Brock-Utne JG, Levitan RM. Laryngoscopy and morbid obesity: a comparison of the "sniff" and "ramped" positions. *Obes Surg* 2004;14:1171–5.

6. Yentis SM, Dob DP. High regional block – the failed intubation of the new millennium? *Int J Obstet Anaesth* 2001;10:159–61.

7. Allman K, McIndoe A, Wilson I (editors). *Emergencies in Anaesthesia*. Second edition. Oxford: Oxford University Press; 2009.

8. Jenkins JG. Some immediate serious complications of obstetric epidural analgesia and anaesthesia: a prospective study of 145,550 epidurals. *Int J Obstet Anest* 2005;14:37–42.

9. National Patient Safety Agency. Patient Safety Alert NPSA/2007/21: Epidural injections and infusions. London: NPSA; 2007 [http://www.nrls.npsa.nhs.uk/resources/?entryid45=59807&q=0%C2%AC2007%2f21%C2%AC].

10. National Patient Safety Agency. Patient Safety Alert NPSA/2009/PSA004B: Safer spinal (intrathecal), epidural and regional devices – Part B. London: NPSA; 2009 [http://www.nrls.npsa.nhs.uk/resources/?entryid45=94529&q=0%C2%ACsafer+spinal%C2%AC].

11. National Patient Safety Agency. Patient Safety Alert NPSA/2009/PSA004A: Safer spinal (intrathecal), epidural and regional devices – Part A (update). London: NPSA; 2011 [http://www.nrls.npsa.nhs.uk/resources/?entryid45=94529&q=0%C2%ACsafer+spinal%C2%AC].

12. Weinberg G, Ripper R, Feinstein DL, Hoffman W. Lipid emulsion infusion rescues dogs from bupivacaine-induced cardiac toxicity. *Reg Anaesth Pain Med* 2003;28:198–202.

13. Rosenblatt MA, Abel M, Fischer GW, Itzkovich CJ, Eisenkraft JB. Successful use of a 20% lipid emulsion to resuscitate a patient after a presumed bupivacaine-related cardiac arrest. *Anesthesiology* 2006;105:217–8.

14. Foxall G, McCahon R, Lamb J, Hardman JG, Bedforth NM. Levobupivacaine-induced seizures and cardiovascular collapse treated with Intralipid. *Anaesthesia* 2007;62:516–8.

Module 5
Fetal monitoring
in labour

Key learning points

■ When performing intermittent auscultation, document fetal heart rate as per NICE guidance, including the frequency, timing and duration (specific to first- and second-stage guidance).

■ To understand the features and terminology of a normal, suspicious and pathological CTG when using electronic fetal monitoring (EFM).

■ To recognise the importance of interpreting the CTG in the context of all clinical circumstances and to propose appropriate actions.

■ It is best practice to record the opinion and action clearly and legibly using a structured pro forma.

■ Specific clinical information in line with national requirements, relevant clinical events and also the CTG opinion should be recorded at the appropriate point on the CTG tracing (in addition to documenting in the partogram).

Problems identified from case discussions

■ Not auscultating the fetal heart simultaneously using a Pinard stethoscope at the start of EFM to confirm the fetal heart rate.

■ Not documenting a systematic assessment of the CTG based on the NICE algorithm at least hourly and at every review.

■ Not involving experienced practitioners to assist with decision making when the CTG is difficult to interpret.

■ Not documenting and signing all relevant actions and CTG opinions on the appropriate section of the CTG in addition to the partogram.

■ Not making an appropriate plan for timely review of the CTG.

■ Not continuing/recommencing EFM until the birth of the baby when delivery is expedited in theatre.

Introduction

Fetal heart rate recording has been a key assessment of fetal health in labour for over 200 years and there are written records as far back as the 17th century describing fetal life; a poem written by Phillipe Le Goust in 1650 refers to hearing the fetal heart 'beating like the clapper of a mill...'. The Pinard stethoscope was introduced in 1876 for performing intermittent auscultation and in 1893 Von Winkel established criteria for determining potential 'fetal distress', some of which criteria are still used today, such as fetal tachycardia over 160 beats/minute, fetal bradycardia less than 100 beats/minute and gross alteration of fetal movements.[1]

Electronic fetal heart rate monitoring (EFM) was first introduced at Yale University in 1958. However, in the UK, it was the late 1960s before EFM began to be used clinically.[2,3] At that time, it was not uncommon for babies to die in labour, apparently with few premonitory signs; therefore, when EFM was first introduced, the original aim was to prevent intrapartum fetal deaths. It was later assumed that EFM would lead to earlier detection of hypoxia, thus allowing timely intervention to reduce cerebral palsy rates.

Meta-analysis of randomised controlled trials of EFM compared with intermittent auscultation have actually shown no difference in perinatal outcome between the two methods, although an increase in operative delivery, particularly caesarean section, has been demonstrated with EFM. However, intervention rates were reduced when fetal blood sampling was used as an adjunct to EFM.[4,5]

It has been suggested that the lack of improvement in perinatal outcome, despite the use of EFM, could be attributable to the insufficient sample size of most randomised trials. Very large studies (35 000 women) would be required to determine the efficacy of EFM. The largest intrapartum fetal monitoring trial, the Dublin trial, found a reduction in neonatal seizures in the EFM arm but no difference in long-term outcome.[6] However, the trial was not large enough to detect differences in the rates of cerebral palsy, as perinatal morbidity and mortality are extremely low. In addition, only about 10% of cerebral palsy cases are related to intrapartum events, as occult infection and/or inflammation are increasingly implicated.[7,8]

It is often forgotten that most randomised trials of EFM and intermittent auscultation have shown that neither method is particularly reliable and there are important 'human' factors that may affect outcome too. Murphy et al. found that, of 64 cases of significant birth asphyxia, abnormalities were missed in both the continuously monitored and intermittent auscultation groups.[9]

Inadequate skill in the interpretation of cardiotocographs (CTGs) and failure to take appropriate action once abnormalities have been detected are key problems. This may have contributed to the failure of EFM to reduce perinatal mortality. These problems have been recurrent themes in many of the reports of the Confidential Enquiry into Stillbirths and Deaths in Infancy (CESDI).[10–12] Grant highlighted that: 'for monitoring to be effective, it must be performed correctly, its results must then be interpreted satisfactorily; and this interpretation must provoke an appropriate response'.[4]

The West Midlands Perinatal Audit found that 70% of intrapartum deaths were considered to have avoidable factors, notably a lack of understanding in CTG interpretation.[12] Consequently, regular training and updates in CTG interpretation have been recommended by CESDI and this has now been implemented in the majority of maternity units in England and Wales.[13]

In 2001, the Royal College of Obstetricians and Gynaecologists produced an evidence-based guideline on fetal monitoring in labour which was subsequently inherited by the National Institute for Health and Clinical Excellence (NICE).[14] The guideline not only aimed to clarify when EFM should be used as an appropriate method for monitoring the fetal heart in labour, but also standardised the classification of CTGs and provided guidance on actions to be taken when abnormalities were detected. This guidance on fetal monitoring in labour was updated in 2008 and is now incorporated within the NICE intrapartum care guideline.[15]

Risk management and training

Both intrapartum death and the birth of a baby with severe brain damage are tragedies to the families concerned. The evidence linking brain injury to intrapartum care is inconsistent but it is a major source of litigation.[16,17] The basis of many claims includes:

- action taken too late
- intermittent auscultation was infrequent
- failure to call medical staff soon enough or often enough.[18]

A Swedish study reviewed the outcomes of infants (over 33 weeks) born in Stockholm County between 2004 and 2006 and found that there was substandard care during labour in two-thirds of infants with a 5-minute Apgar score of less than 7. The main reasons for the substandard care were related to misinterpretation of the CTG, not acting on a pathological CTG in a timely fashion, and imprudent use of oxytocin.[19]

If care is found to be suboptimal, this is likely to be indefensible in court and individual claims can exceed £3 million. Adequate interpretation of CTGs is crucial to quality improvement and the reduction of medico-legal risk. In the UK, claims for damaged babies account for 50% of the NHS litigation bill.[20]

All practitioners involved in intrapartum care should ensure that they have the knowledge and skills to interpret CTGs and act appropriately, with the aim of providing high-quality, defensible care. The Clinical Negligence Scheme for Trusts (CNST) Maternity Standards mandate that individual maternity units should have a training needs analysis which includes regular fetal monitoring training for all relevant staff in line with national recommendations.[21]

Draycott et al. have demonstrated that mandatory skills training in CTG interpretation and obstetric emergencies has improved neonatal outcomes in one UK maternity unit, and the Northern California Kaiser Permanente Perinatal Patient Safety Program described an improved safety climate after training.[22,23] The training covered not only CTG interpretation but also the skills required to communicate the interpretation and the actions of the team responding to the emergency, indicating that improving outcomes in labour when EFM is used is probably dependent on more than just CTG interpretation training alone. A recent systematic review by Pehrson at al. concluded that training can improve CTG competence and clinical practice, but further research is needed to evaluate the type and content of training that is most effective.[24]

Physiology and pathophysiology

The healthy fetus is able to cope with the stresses of labour and adapts appropriately to meet the challenge. The current evidence base supports the use of intermittent auscultation for 'low-risk' mothers.

Fetal oxygen supply

In comparison with adults, the fetal partial pressure of oxygen is relatively low; however, the fetus has a remarkable margin of safety. A high concentration of fetal haemoglobin and its greater affinity for absorbing oxygen means that oxygen saturation is high. The cardiac output of the fetus is also extremely efficient. Consequently, the fetal oxygen supply is usually greater than requirements.

Gas exchange is impaired during contractions, which means that oxygen levels fall and carbon dioxide (CO_2) levels rise. Between contractions the oxygen supply is restored and the accumulated CO_2 is excreted.

Conditions that impair gas exchange at the placenta, such as uterine hypercontractility, cord occlusion, maternal hypotension or abruption, will cause retention of CO_2, which lowers the pH of the fetal blood (a respiratory acidosis). This should be resolved when placental perfusion is restored. However, if gas exchange continues to be impeded, the fetus will rely on the following important defence mechanisms:

■ **Hormonal response**

A reduction in fetal oxygen supply is detected by chemoreceptors in the fetal aorta. This activates a hormonal response with an increase in catecholamines, vasopressin, adenine and adenosine levels. The levels of catecholamines in an asphyxiated infant exceed those of patients with phaeochromocytoma.[25]

■ **Preferential redistribution of blood flow**

There is a decrease in blood flow to less 'essential' organs such as the liver, spleen, gut, kidneys and skin. Blood supply to the 'priority' organs – brain, heart and adrenal glands – is increased. The heart needs to work harder during this time and myocardial blood flow can increase up to 500% in response to hypoxia. Oxygen requirements for the brain are not as great and fetal behaviour can adapt to reduce energy requirements.

■ **Glycogenolysis**

When the oxygen supply is no longer sufficient to meet the energy requirements of the fetus, glycogenolysis is activated by the hormonal response. This means that glucose is released from glycogen stores and is metabolised anaerobically (without oxygen) to maintain energy requirements. Release of adrenaline stimulates the activation of glycogenolysis.

During anaerobic metabolism, stores of glycogen in the heart, muscle and liver are broken down to provide energy. Lactic acid, a by-product of anaerobic metabolism, is initially buffered (neutralised) but will eventually cause the pH of the blood to fall further (metabolic acidosis). As the fetus continues to use glycogen stores, the acidosis becomes predominantly metabolic in origin and the pH decreases even further.

Clearly, conditions and events that affect the mother (pre-eclampsia, diabetes, antepartum haemorrhage) and/or placental function (too frequent or prolonged uterine contractions) and/or the baby's defence mechanisms (growth restriction, infection, chronic hypoxaemia and stress) may make the fetus less able to adapt and more vulnerable to hypoxia (Box 5.1).

Box 5.1 Factors that influence fetal oxygenation

Mother	Uterus/placenta	Fetus
Anaemia	Abruption	Anaemia
Analgesia/anaesthesia	Cord prolapse	Fetal bleeding
Dehydration	Impaired placental function	Infection
Hypertension	Uterine hypercontractility	Growth restriction
Hypotension		
Pyrexia		

Compensatory responses and adaptation to hypoxia can protect the fetus for only a finite amount of time. When the defence mechanisms are blunted, depleted or overwhelmed, the risk of perinatal asphyxia (hypoxia, acidosis and tissue damage) is increased.

Standards and quality

The indications for offering women continuous EFM in labour have been documented in the NICE intrapartum care guideline,[15] which should be implemented locally and available on every labour ward. The guideline recommends that risk factors should be recorded in the mother's notes as part of the admission assessment, together with appropriate action plans (Figure 5.1).[15]

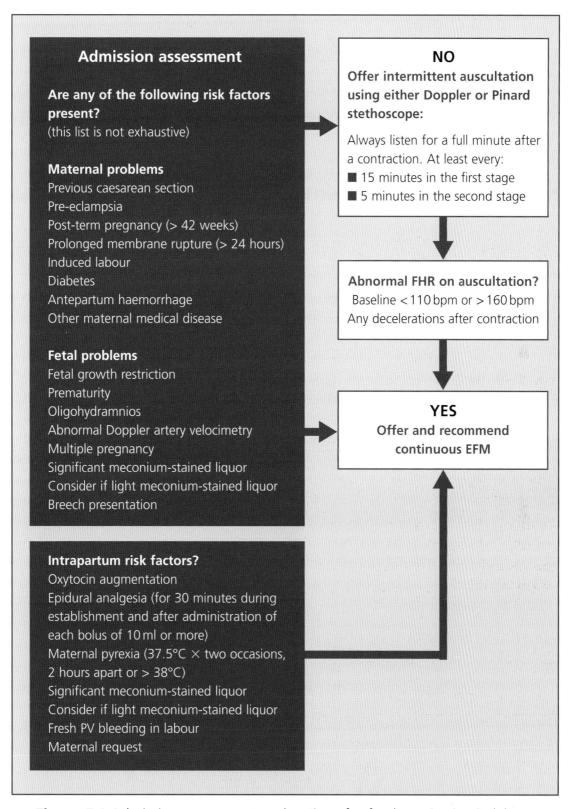

Figure 5.1 Admission assessment and options for fetal monitoring in labour (based on NICE Guidelines 2001 and 2007)[14,15]

Informed choice

The assessment of fetal wellbeing is only one aspect of intrapartum care. It is important that attention is given to an informed choice based on the available evidence. An information leaflet, 'Monitoring your baby's heartbeat in labour: information for pregnant women', is available for download from the NICE website.[26]

Standards for intermittent auscultation in labour

For a mother who is healthy and has an uncomplicated pregnancy, intermittent auscultation should be offered and recommended in labour using either a Doppler ultrasound or a Pinard stethoscope, to monitor fetal wellbeing.[15]

In the active stages of labour:

- First stage of labour: intermittent auscultation should occur at least every 15 minutes, after a contraction, and for a minimum of 60 seconds. Count the fetal heart rate over a full minute and record the rate on the partogram.[27]

- Second stage of labour: intermittent auscultation should occur every 5 minutes, after a contraction, and for a minimum of 60 seconds.

- Any intrapartum events that may affect the fetal heart rate should be noted contemporaneously in the maternal notes, signed and the time noted.

- If a fetal heart rate abnormality is suspected, the maternal pulse should be palpated simultaneously with the fetal heart to differentiate between the two heart rates.

Continuous EFM should be offered and recommended when:

- a baseline of less than 110 beats/minute or greater than 160 beats/minute is heard during intermittent auscultation

- any decelerations are suspected after a contraction

- any intrapartum risk factors develop (Figure 5.1; page 63).

The current evidence base does not support the use of the admission CTG in low-risk pregnancies and is therefore not recommended.[15]

Technical considerations for EFM in labour

It is best to auscultate the fetal heart using a Pinard stethoscope before commencing EFM in labour. In addition, the maternal pulse should be palpated regularly with any form of fetal monitoring, to differentiate between maternal and fetal heart rates. It is possible to generate a signal from a large pulsating maternal vessel, which may be misinterpreted as the fetal heart. Also, the ultrasound may falsely double the rate of the maternal pulse if there is sufficient extended separation between valve movements, generating a rate that would be within the normal range of the fetal heart.

There have been occasional reports of unexpected macerated stillbirths with apparently normal intrapartum CTGs, even with direct fetal scalp clip application.[28,29] It is therefore important that, if fetal death is suspected (despite the presence of an apparently recorded fetal heart rate), fetal viability should be confirmed with real-time ultrasound assessment.

All members of staff should be aware of the technical limitations of EFM and should always read the manufacturer's instructions for each particular monitor.

Standards for electronic fetal monitoring

EFM should not be used as a tool of convenience in place of skilled midwives when monitoring the fetal heart in labour. The unselected use of continuous EFM contributes to unnecessary intervention.

- The date and time clocks on the machine should be correct and paper speed set to 1 cm/minute (Figure 5.2).
- CTGs should be labelled with the mother's name and hospital number and dated (Figure 5.2).
- Any intrapartum events that may affect the fetal heart rate should be noted contemporaneously on the CTG, signed and dated (such as vaginal examinations, fetal blood sampling, epidural insertion and top-ups).
- If external monitoring is not of sufficient quality for interpretation of the CTG, a fetal scalp electrode should be applied where possible.
- Any consultations should be documented in the case notes and on the CTG, together with the date, time and signature.
- Following the birth, the caregiver should sign and note the date, time and mode of delivery on the CTG (Figure 5.2).
- The CTG should be stored securely with the maternal notes.

CTG check list (attach to start of CTG trace)		
Reason for CTG:		
Date:	Date set correctly on CTG? (tick)	
Time:	Time set correctly on CTG? (tick)	
Name:	Paper speed set to 1cm per min (tick)	
Hospital number:	Gestation:	
	Maternal pulse (rate):	
(or attach addressograph)	FH auscultated prior to CTG (rate):	

Attach to end of CTG trace	
Mode of birth:	Date of birth:
Signature:	Time of birth:

Figure 5.2 Example of start and end stickers for attaching to CTG

Features of the intrapartum CTG and terminology

Most clinicians would have no difficulty in recognising the features of a normal intrapartum CTG, as shown in Figure 5.3. However, it is important to remember that a suspicious or pathological CTG does not necessarily mean the fetus is hypoxic (insufficient oxygen to meet requirements). In fact, often this is not the case, as illustrated in Figure 5.4. When the CTG is normal, we can be confident that the fetus will be normoxic, so the sensitivity of the CTG is high. However, when the CTG is pathological or suspicious, only about 50% of fetuses will show some degree of hypoxia, so its specificity is low; hence the need for a further test in the form of fetal blood sampling whenever possible and if appropriate.

In addition, there is no reliable way to determine fetal reserves or, often, the nature or severity of the event. The growth-restricted fetus may have a blunted response owing to chronic stress and inadequate glycogen stores. Acute catastrophic events may quickly overwhelm the defence mechanisms

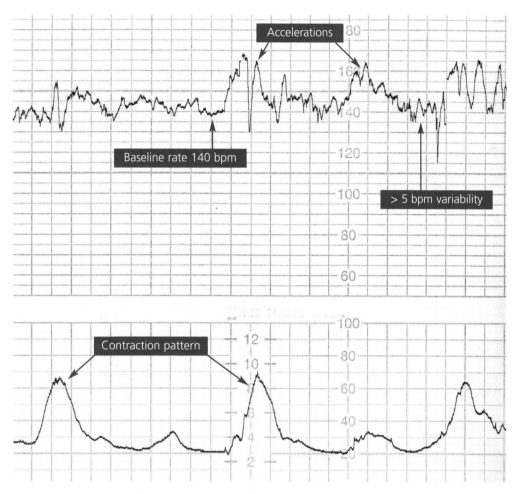

Figure 5.3 Normal intrapartum CTG

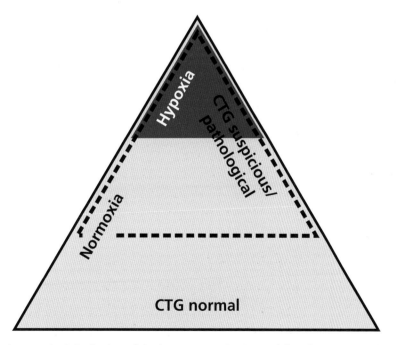

Figure 5.4 Relationship between CTG and fetal oxygenation

of even a healthy baby. The CTG must thus always be interpreted in the context of the antepartum and intrapartum clinical history and events.

Clearly, it is important that communication between carers should convey the clinical context using consistent terminology to describe the features of the intrapartum CTG, the level of concern and the urgency of the situation.

There are four main features that should be systematically examined to assist with the interpretation of the CTG:

- baseline rate
- baseline variability
- accelerations
- decelerations.

These features, in conjunction with the contraction pattern and the clinical circumstances, should all be considered when deciding the action to be taken.

Baseline fetal heart rate

Baseline fetal heart rate is the level of the fetal heart rate when it is stable, excluding accelerations and decelerations. It is determined over a time period of 5 or 10 minutes and expressed in beats/minute (see Figure 5.3). The ranges and descriptive terms are shown in Table 5.1.

Table 5.1 Baseline ranges

Level	Rate (beats/minute)
Reassuring	
Normal baseline	110–160
Non-reassuring	
Moderate bradycardia	100–109
Moderate tachycardia[a]	161–180
Abnormal	
Abnormal bradycardia	<100
Abnormal tachycardia	>180

[a] A tachycardia of 161–180 beats/minute, where accelerations are present and no other adverse features appear, should NOT be regarded as suspicious. However, an increase in the baseline rate, even within the normal range, with other non-reassuring or abnormal features should increase concern[14]

Baseline variability

Baseline variability is the minor fluctuation in baseline fetal heart rate occurring at three to five cycles/minute (see Figure 5.3).

Normal baseline variability:	Greater than or equal to 5 beats/minute between contractions for up to 40 minutes.
Non-reassuring baseline variability:	Less than 5 beats/minute for 40 minutes or more but less than 90 minutes.
Abnormal baseline variability:	Less than 5 beats/minute for 90 minutes or more.

Note: if repeated accelerations are present with reduced variability, this should be regarded as a reassuring feature and should be taken into consideration when deciding the opinion of the CTG.[15]

Accelerations

Accelerations are an abrupt transient increase in the fetal heart rate of 15 beats/minute or more, lasting 15 seconds or more (Figure 5.3). The absence of accelerations with an otherwise normal CTG is of uncertain significance.

Decelerations

Decelerations are a transient slowing of the fetal heart rate below the baseline level of 15 beats/minute or more for a period of 15 seconds or more.

Early decelerations:	Uniform, repetitive, periodic slowing of the fetal heart rate with onset early in the contraction and return to baseline at the end of the contraction. The lowest point of the deceleration will coincide with the highest point of the contraction. Early decelerations are usually associated with head compression and hence tend to occur late in the first stage or during the second stage of labour. True uniform early decelerations are rare and benign and are therefore not significant and not associated with fetal hypoxia.
Late decelerations:	Uniform, repetitive, periodic slowing of the fetal heart rate with onset mid- to end of the contraction and lowest point more than 20 seconds after the peak of the contraction, always

ending after the contraction. In the presence of a non-accelerative trace with baseline variability less than 5 beats/minute, the definition would include decelerations less than 15 beats/minute. Late decelerations, if present for more than 30 minutes,* are indicative of fetal hypoxia and further action is indicated (Figure 5.5).[15]

* It may not be appropriate to wait 30 minutes to refer for obstetric review if the CTG is showing late decelerations from the start of the tracing.

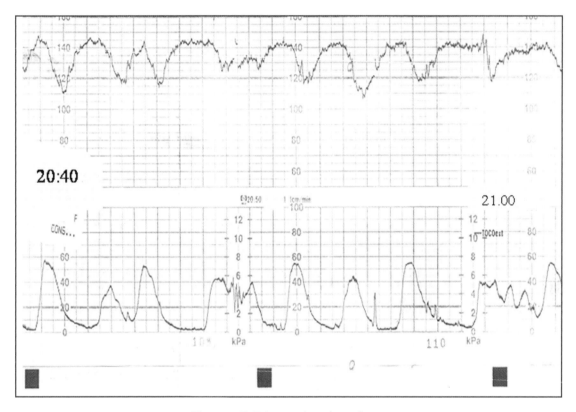

Figure 5.5 Late decelerations

Variable decelerations:

These are the most common form of deceleration occurring during labour. A variable, intermittent periodic slowing of the fetal heart rate, with rapid onset and recovery. Time relationships with contraction cycle are variable and they occur in isolation. Sometimes they resemble other types of deceleration patterns in timing and shape. They are often caused by compression of the umbilical cord, and can be typical or atypical (Figure 5.6). Typical variable decelerations are an autonomic nervous system response to cord compression and are indicative of the fetus coping well in labour.

However, the fetus may become tired over time and, if decelerations occur with more than 50% of contractions for more than 90 minutes,* this should be regarded as non- reassuring, particularly if there is any degree of fetal compromise such as fetal growth restriction.[16] Atypical variable decelerations may subsequently develop, indicating that the fetus is now less able to cope with the cord compression.

*It may not be appropriate to wait 90 minutes (typical variable) or 30 minutes (atypical variable) to refer for obstetric review if the CTG is showing typical or atypical variable decelerations from the start of the tracing.

Atypical variable decelerations:	Variable decelerations with any of the following components (Figure 5.6):

■ loss of primary or secondary rise in baseline rate (shouldering)

■ slow return to baseline fetal heart rate after the end of the contraction

■ prolonged secondary rise in baseline rate (exaggerated shouldering)

■ a biphasic deceleration

■ loss of variability during deceleration

■ continuation of baseline rate at lower level.

If atypical variable decelerations occur with more than 50% of contractions for more than 30 minutes, they should be defined as abnormal; the CTG is therefore pathological, indicating that further action is required.[15]

Prolonged deceleration:	An abrupt decrease in the fetal heart rate to levels below the baseline that lasts for up to 120 seconds. If a fetal bradycardia occurs for more than 3 minutes, plans should be made to urgently expedite birth using the most appropriate method. A 'category 1 birth' should be declared and the woman should be transferred to theatre immediately. If the fetal heart recovers within

Electronic Fetal Monitoring in Labour

Variable decelerations

Variable decelerations are the most common form of deceleration occurring during labour.

Definition: A variable, intermittent, periodic slowing of the fetal heart rate with rapid onset and recovery. Time relationships with contraction cycle are variable and they occur in isolation. Sometimes they resemble other types of deceleration patterns in timing and shape. They are often caused by compression of the umbilical cord, and can be typical or atypical.

Typical variable decelerations are an autonomic nervous system response to cord compression and are indicative of the fetus coping well with the cord compression. However, the fetus may become tired over time and, if they occur with more than 50% of contractions for more than 90 minutes, this should be regarded as non-reassuring, particularly if there is any degree of fetal compromise such as intrauterine growth restriction.

Atypical variable decelerations may subsequently develop indicating that the fetus is now less able to cope with the cord compression.

Atypical variable decelerations may have any of the following components:
- Loss of primary or secondary rise in baseline rate (shouldering)
- Slow return to baseline FHR after the end of the contraction
- Prolonged secondary rise in baseline rate (exaggerated shouldering)
- A biphasic deceleration
- Loss of variability during deceleration
- Continuation of baseline rate at lower level.

> **If atypical variable decelerations occur with more than 50% of contractions for over 30 minutes, they should be defined as abnormal and the CTG is therefore pathological, indicating that further action is required.**

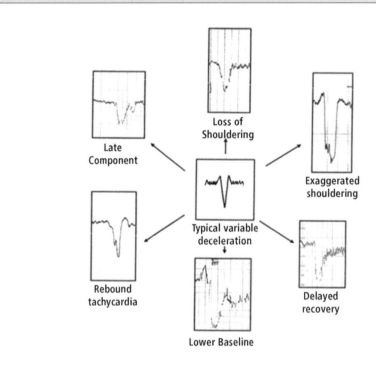

Figure 5.6 Poster displaying typical and atypical variable decelerations

9 minutes, the decision for immediate delivery should be reconsidered if reasonable, and in consultation with the woman.

Sinusoidal pattern: A regular oscillation of the baseline long-term variability resembling a sine wave. This undulating pattern, lasting at least 10 minutes, has a relatively fixed period of 3–5 cycles/minute and an amplitude of 5–15 beats/minute above and below the baseline. Baseline variability is absent. A true sinusoidal pattern is an abnormal feature and is associated with high rates of fetal morbidity and mortality (Figure 5.7).[30]

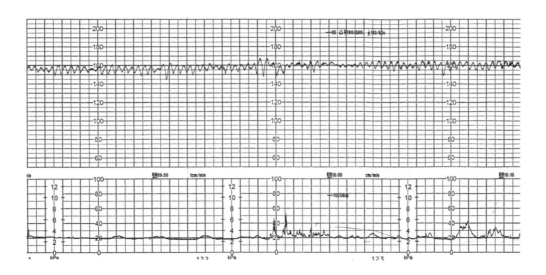

Figure 5.7 Sinusoidal pattern

Contraction pattern: Always remember to look at the 'bottom line'. Take notice of the duration of contractions and the interval between contractions, observing for signs of hypercontractility, or frequent, low-amplitude contractions in association with a suspicious or pathological CTG that may be suggestive of placental abruption.

Interpretation of the intrapartum CTG

Having considered and observed the four main features of the CTG, the trace should be classified as normal, suspicious or pathological, depending on the presence of any non-reassuring or abnormal features.

The clinical circumstances should always be considered when deciding actions to be taken if a CTG is classified as suspicious or pathological in labour. A structured CTG pro forma (based on the NICE intrapartum care guideline), which incorporates relevant guidance on CTG interpretation in a single implementation tool, can be used to not only document the four main features and classify the CTG, but also to record actions that should be taken.[15] Figure 5.8 is an example of an intrapartum CTG pro forma that incorporates all of the NICE guidance for CTG interpretation.

Intrapartum CTG Proforma	Reassuring (Acceptable)	Non-reassuring	Abnormal	North Bristol NHS
Baseline rate (bpm)	110 – 160 Rate:	100 – 109 Rate: 161 – 180 Rate:	Less than 100 Rate: More than 180 Rate: Sinusoidal pattern for 10 minutes or more	Comments:-
N.B Rising baseline rate even within normal range may be of concern if other non-reassuring / abnormal features present.				
Variability (bpm)	5 bpm or more	Less than 5 bpm for 40 - 90 minutes	Less than 5 bpm for 90 minutes	Comments:-
Accelerations	Present	None for 40 mins	Comments	
Decelerations	None	Typical variable decelerations with more than 50% of contractions for more than 90 minutes	Atypical variable decelerations with more than 50% of contractions for more than 30 minutes	Comments:-
	Typical variable decelerations with more than 50% of contractions but for less than 90 minutes	Atypical variable decelerations with more than 50% of contractions for less than 30 minutes	Late decelerations for more than 30 minutes	
	Typical or atypical variable decelerations with less than 50% of contractions	Late decelerations for less than 30 minutes		
	True early decelerations	Single prolonged deceleration for up to 3 minutes	Single prolonged deceleration for more than 3 minutes	
N.B If CTG has any non-reassuring or abnormal features present from commencement of monitoring, it may not be appropriate to wait 30 or 90 minutes before requesting review				
Opinion	Normal CTG (All 4 features reassuring)	Suspicious CTG (1 non-reassuring feature)	Pathological CTG (2 or more non-reassuring or 1 or more abnormal features)	
Cont's: :10	Maternal pulse:	Liquor colour:	Dilatation (cm):	Gestation (wks):
Action:				
Date:	Time:	Signature:............................Print:............................Designation:............		

Figure 5.8 An example of an intrapartum CTG pro forma that incorporates all of the NICE guidance for CTG interpretation

Suspicious CTG

An intrapartum CTG with one non-reassuring feature is classified as suspicious. Figure 5.9 shows the NICE guideline's suggested actions when the CTG is suspicious.

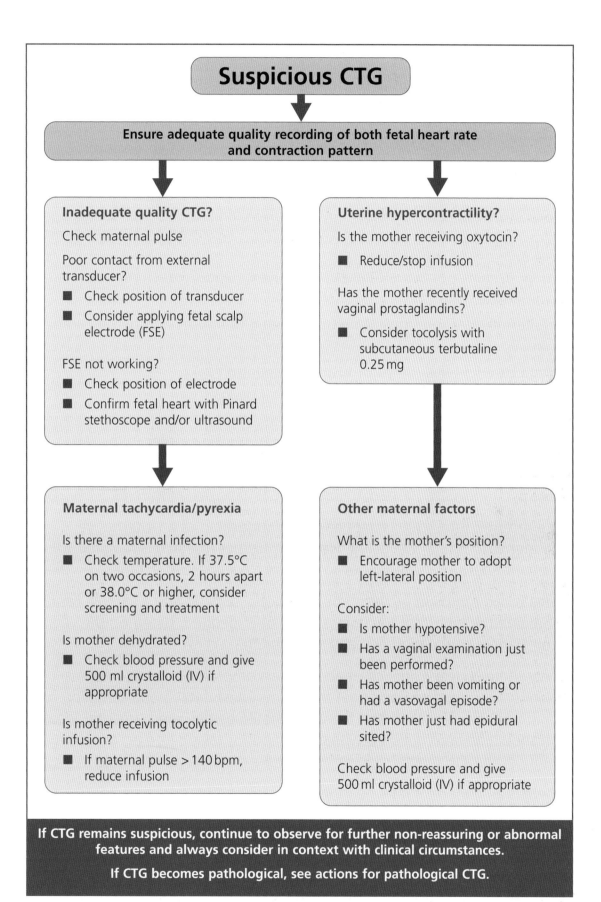

Figure 5.9 Suggested actions if CTG suspicious

Pathological CTG and fetal blood sampling

An intrapartum CTG with two or more non-reassuring features or one or more abnormal features is classified as pathological. When considering expediting birth because of a pathological CTG, it is recommended that fetal blood sampling be performed prior to intervening (in the absence of technical difficulties or contraindications) to determine the presence and extent of fetal acidosis. Therefore, maternity units that employ EFM should have ready access to fetal blood sampling facilities.

Contraindications include:

- clear evidence of acute fetal compromise in labour which requires immediate action
- maternal infection (for example HIV, hepatitis viruses and herpes simplex virus)
- fetal bleeding disorders (for example haemophilia)
- prematurity (gestational age less than 34 weeks).

Fetal blood sampling should be undertaken with the mother in the left-lateral position.

Figure 5.10 shows suggested actions if the CTG is pathological.[15]

More recently, fetal scalp lactate has been suggested as an alternative measurement of fetal wellbeing. However, further research is required to determine specific lactate ranges in relation to neonatal outcomes.

If fetal blood sampling proves to be technically difficult and a sample cannot be obtained, the birth of the baby should be expedited, based on the clinical circumstances of the mother, baby and the CTG.

Where there is clear evidence of acute fetal compromise (for example, a prolonged deceleration for longer than 3 minutes), fetal blood sampling should not be undertaken and the baby should be delivered urgently. Ideally, birth should be accomplished within 30 minutes, taking into account the severity of the situation.

If there is an abnormal fetal heart rate pattern and uterine hypercontractility which is not secondary to the use of an oxytocin infusion, tocolysis should be considered. The suggested regimen is subcutaneous terbutaline 0.25 mg.[15] Its use may also be considered to reduce uterine activity and aid in utero resuscitation when preparing for a category 1 birth. If terbutaline is used, anticipate the possibility of uterine atony post-birth and treat accordingly.

Pathological CTG

Fetal blood sampling (FBS) possible and/or appropriate?

Encourage mother to adopt left-lateral position. Check blood pressure and give 500 ml crystalloid (IV) if appropriate.

FBS result (pH)	Recommended action
Normal 7.25 or above	– FBS should be repeated in 1 hour if FHR abnormality persists or sooner if there are further abnormalities – If result remains stable after second test, a third/further sample may be deferred unless there are further abnormalities of the CTG
Borderline 7.21–7.24	– Repeat FBS within 30 minutes if the FHR remains pathological or sooner if there are further abnormalities (consideration should be given to the time taken to perform FBS when planning repeat samples) – If a third sample is indicated, a consultant obstetric opinion should be sought
Abnormal 7.20 or less	– Consultant obstetric advice should be sought – Expedite birth within 30 minutes

All FBS results should be interpreted taking into account the previous pH measurement, the rate of progress in labour and the clinical features of mother and fetus.

Fetal blood sampling not possible/inappropriate?

– Encourage mother to adopt left-lateral position. Check blood pressure and give 500 ml crystalloid (IV) if appropriate.

EXPEDITE BIRTH:

– The urgency and mode of birth should take into account the severity of the fetal heart rate and the clinical circumstances.

– The accepted standard is that birth should be accomplished within 30 minutes.

Figure 5.10 Suggested actions if CTG pathological

Adverse effects of terbutaline include maternal tachycardia (palpitations) and, hence, fetal tachycardia may occur. Raised blood pressure, tremor, nausea, nervousness and dizziness may also occur.

Continuous EFM in the presence of oxytocin

If the fetal heart rate is normal and an oxytocin infusion is required during labour, a full assessment by an experienced midwife or obstetrician (depending on the parity of the woman) should be performed and documented in the maternal labour notes. The oxytocin infusion may be increased until the woman is experiencing four or five contractions every 10 minutes. The infusion rate should be reduced if contractions occur more frequently than five contractions in 10 minutes.

If the fetal heart rate trace is classified as suspicious when an oxytocin infusion is in progress, review by an experienced obstetrician should be requested. Once reviewed, the obstetrician may recommend that the oxytocin continues to be increased but only to a dose which achieves four to five contractions in 10 minutes.[15]

If the fetal heart rate trace is classified as pathological, the oxytocin infusion should be stopped and a full assessment of the fetal condition should be undertaken by an experienced obstetrician. Consideration may be given to re-starting the oxytocin based on the findings of the fetal assessment.

The prolonged use of maternal facial oxygen therapy may be harmful to the fetus and should therefore be avoided. There is also currently no evidence evaluating the benefits or risks associated with the short-term use of maternal facial oxygen therapy in cases of suspected fetal compromise. However, the anaesthetist may request facial oxygen to be administered purely for maternal pre-oxygenation before an operative procedure.

Newborn assessment

The Apgar score, need for intubation and abnormal behaviour are important components of the assessment of the newborn baby. However, they are subjective, provide incomplete information and are not by themselves indicative of asphyxia. In the perinatal period, asphyxia is defined as the combination of hypoxia and acidosis with impaired organ function.[31] Thus, both clinical and biochemical information are required to differentiate between an asphyxiated infant and one that is depressed for other reasons (infection, congenital abnormalities or maternal analgesia). Paired blood samples from the umbilical artery and umbilical vein should be collected to provide an objective outcome measure. The RCOG recommends that paired samples should be obtained as a minimum when:

- emergency caesarean section is performed
- instrumental vaginal birth is performed
- shoulder dystocia has occurred
- fetal blood sampling has been performed in labour
- the baby's condition is poor at birth with an Apgar score of 6 or less at 5 minutes.

The umbilical cord acid–base status at time of birth can be important for medico-legal reasons and for risk management strategies.[32] Clamped cord segments or blood stored in syringes can be left at room temperature for up to 60 minutes without significant changes in pH or CO_2.[33,34]

Antenatal CTG interpretation

Although the evidence for EFM use antenatally is based on only a few small studies (four trials and 1588 women in total) from the 1980s, when CTG monitoring was just being introduced into routine clinical practice, a systematic review in the *Cochrane Database of Systematic Reviews* did not confirm or refute any benefits of routine CTG monitoring of 'at risk' pregnancies.[35]

In clinical practice, there are a variety of antenatal indications for undertaking a CTG from 26 weeks of gestation onwards. The presence of a normal fetal heart rate pattern (i.e. showing accelerations of fetal heart rate coinciding with fetal movements) is indicative of a healthy fetus with a properly functioning autonomic nervous system.

The RCOG Green-top Guideline on the management of reduced fetal movements recommends that interpretation of the antenatal CTG fetal heart rate pattern can be assisted by adopting the NICE classification of fetal heart rate features as indicated in their intrapartum care guideline.[36] Therefore, as is the case when classifying intrapartum CTGs, it would seem reasonable to use a structured pro forma to ensure the use of consistent terminology. However, using an intrapartum pro forma is not appropriate as it acknowledges that some decelerations are acceptable in labour, which clearly cannot be the case for antenatal CTGs where there are no contractions. It is also important to remember that the reason for performing an antenatal CTG is particularly relevant when determining any action to be taken, as is the gestation and the status of the membranes.

Figure 5.11 is an example of an antenatal CTG pro forma that may be used for the classification of CTGs in non-labouring women only.

Antenatal CTG Proforma	Reassuring	Non-reassuring	North Bristol **NHS** NHS Trust		
Baseline rate (bpm)	110 – 160 Rate:	Less than 109 Rate: More than 161 Rate: Sinusoidal pattern for 10 mins or more	Comments:-		
N.B Rising baseline rate even within normal range may be of concern if other non-reassuring features present					
Variability (bpm)	5 bpm or more	Less than 5 bpm for more than 40 minutes	Comments:-		
Accelerations	Present	None for 40 mins	Comments		
Decelerations	None	Unprovoked deceleration/s Decelerations related to uterine tightenings (not in labour)	Comments:-		
Opinion	*Normal CTG* (All 4 features reassuring)	*Abnormal CTG* (1or more non-reassuring features)			
	Maternal pulse:	Membranes ruptured: Y / N If yes, date and time:	Liquor colour:	Gestation (wks):	
Reason for CTG:					
Action: (An abnormal CTG requires prompt review by experienced obstetrician/senior midwife)					
Date:	Time:	Signature:...........................Print:............................Designation:.....................			

Figure 5.11 An example of an antenatal CTG pro forma

Antenatal CTG classification

Normal: A CTG where all four features fall into the 'reassuring' category.

Abnormal: A CTG with any non-reassuring features (including any decelerations).

When an abnormal CTG is identified, it should be reviewed by an experienced obstetrician as soon as possible (within 30 minutes) to make a clear individualised action plan, to include:

■ other tests to be performed (ultrasound scan for growth, Doppler studies, etc.)

■ a specified time for the next obstetric review

■ consideration for expediting birth.

Pre-course electronic fetal monitoring CTG workbook

A pre-course CTG workbook will be provided by your course tutor. Participants should complete the workbook before the course and should be ready to discuss the cases on the day of the course. The cases will be reviewed and discussed in small group sessions. The workbooks will not be scored or marked in any way.

References

1. elearning for health. RCOG/RCM EFM training package. 2011.

2. Hon EH. The electronic evaluation of the fetal heart rate; preliminary report. *Am J Obstet Gynecol* 1958;75:1215–30.

3. Beard RW, Filshie GM, Knight CA, Roberts GM. The significance of the changes in the continuous fetal heart rate in the first stage of labour. *J Obstet Gynaecol Br Commonw* 1971;78:865–81.

4. Grant A. Monitoring the fetus during labour. In: Chalmers I, Enkin M, Keirse MC (editors). *A Guide to Effective Care in Pregnancy and Childbirth*. Oxford: Oxford University Press; 1989. p. 846–82.

5. Thacker SB, Stroup D, Chang M. Continuous electronic heart rate monitoring for fetal assessment during labor. *Cochrane Database Syst Rev* 2001;(2):CD000063.

6. MacDonald D, Grant A, Sheridan-Pereira M, Boylan P, Chalmers I. The Dublin randomized controlled trial of intrapartum fetal heart rate monitoring. *Am J Obstet Gynecol* 1985;152:524–39.

7. Nelson KB. What proportion of cerebral palsy is related to birth asphyxia? *J Pediatr* 1988;112:572–4.

8. Nelson KB, Willoughby RE. Infection, inflammation, and the risk of cerebral palsy. *Curr Opin Neurol* 2000;13:133–9.

9. Murphy KW, Johnson P, Moorcraft J, Pattison R, Russell V, Turnbull A. Birth asphyxia and the intrapartum cardiotocograph. *Br J Obstet Gynaecol* 1990;97:470–9.

10. Confidential Enquiry into Stillbirths and Deaths in Infancy. *4th Annual Report*. London: Maternal and Child Health Research Consortium; 1997.

11. Confidential Enquiry into Stillbirths and Deaths in Infancy. *5th Annual Report*. London: Maternal and Child Health Research Consortium; 1998.

12. Confidential Enquiry into Stillbirths and Deaths in Infancy. *7th Annual Report*. London: Maternal and Child Health Research Consortium; 2001.

13. West Midlands Perinatal Audit. Stillbirth and Neonatal Death 1991–1994. Report of National, Regional, District and Unit Mortality Rates. Keele: West Midlands Perinatal Audit; 1996.

14. Royal College of Obstetricians and Gynaecologists. *Electronic Fetal Monitoring*. National Evidence-based Clinical Guideline. London: RCOG Press; 2001.

15. National Collaborating Centre for Women's and Children's Health. *Intrapartum care: care of healthy women and their babies during childbirth*. NICE cinical guideline 55. London: RCOG Press; 2007.

16. Clements RV, Simanowitz A. Cerebral palsy: the international consensus statement. *Clin Risk* 2000;6:135–6.

17. Pickering J. Legal comment on the international consensus statement on causation of cerebral palsy. *Clin Risk* 2000;6:143–4.

18. Symonds EM. Litigation and birth related injuries. In: Chamberlain G (editor). *How to Avoid Medico-legal Problems in Obstetrics and Gynaecology*. London: Chameleon Press; 1991.

19. Berglund S, Pettersson H, Cnattingius S, Grunewald C. How often is a low Apgar score the result of substandard care during labour? *BJOG* 2010;117:968–78.

20. The NHS Litigation Authority. Factsheet 3: information on claims. London: NHSLA; 2011 [http://www.nhsla.com].

21. NHS Litigation Authority. Clinical Negligence Scheme for Trusts Maternity Clinical Risk Management Standards. London: NHSLA; 2011 [http://www.nhsla.com/RiskManagement/].

22. Draycott T, Sibanda T, Owen L, Akande V, Winter C, Reading S, et al. Does training in obstetric emergencies improve neonatal outcome? *BJOG* 2006;113:177–82.

23. MacEachin SR, Lopez CM, Powell KJ, Corbett NL. The fetal heart rate collaborative practice project: situational awareness in electronic fetal monitoring – A Kaiser Permanente Perinatal Patient Safety Program Initiative. *J Perinat Neonatal Nurs* 2009;23:314–23.

24. Pehrson C, Sorensen J, Amer-Wåhlin I. Evaluation and impact of cardiotocography training programmes: a systematic review. *BJOG* 2011;118:926–35.

25. Lagercrantz H, Bistoletti P. Catecholamine release in the newborn infant at birth. *Pediatr Res* 1977;11:889–93.

26. National Institute for Health and Clinical Excellence. *Monitoring your baby's heartbeat in labour. A Guide for Patients and their Carers*. London: NICE; 2001 [www.nice.org.uk/nicemedia/pdf/efmpatleafenglish.pdf].

27. The Map of Medicine: Evidence Summary for the First Stage of Labour. International. 2011 [http://eng.mapofmedicine.com/evidence/map/normal_birth1.html].

28. Herbert WN, Stuart NN, Butler LS. Electronic fetal heart rate monitoring with intrauterine fetal demise. *J Obstet Gynecol Neonatal Nurs* 1987;16:249–52.

29. Maeder HP, Lippert TH. Misinterpretation of heart rate recordings in fetal death. *Eur J Obstet Gynecol* 1972;6:167–70.

30. Schneider EP, Tropper PJ. The variable deceleration, prolonged deceleration, and sinusoidal fetal heart rate. *Clin Obstet Gynecol* 1986;29:64–72.

31. Greene KR, Rosen KG. Intrapartum asphyxia. In: Levene MI, Lilford R (editors). *Fetal and Neonatal Neurology and Neurosurgery*. Second edition. Edinburgh: Churchill Livingstone; 1995. p. 389–404.

32. MacLennan A. A template for defining a causal relation between acute intrapartum events and cerebral palsy: international consensus statement. *BMJ* 1999;319:1054–9.

33. Duerbeck NB, Chaffin DG, Seeds JW. A practical approach to umbilical artery pH and blood gas determinations. *Obstet Gynecol* 1992;79:959–62.

34. Sykes GS, Molloy PM. Effects of delays in collection or analysis on the results of umbilical cord blood measurements. *Br J Obstet Gynaecol* 1984;91:989–92.

35. Pattison N, McCowan L. Cardiotocography for antepartum fetal assessment. *Cochrane Database Syst Rev* 2000;(2):CD001068.

36. Royal College of Obstetricians and Gynaecologists. *Reduced fetal movements*. Green-top Guideline No. 57. London: RCOG; 2011 [http://www.rcog.org.uk/womens-health/clinical-guidance/reduced-fetal-movements-green-top-57].

Module 6
Pre-eclampsia and eclampsia

Key learning points

- To understand the risk factors and recognise the signs and symptoms of severe pre-eclampsia.

- To understand the potential complications of severe hypertension (systolic blood pressure $\geq$160 mmHg) and its management.

- To manage an eclamptic seizure effectively.

- To understand the care and monitoring required when a woman is being treated with magnesium sulphate.

- The importance of detailed contemporaneous documentation.

Common difficulties observed in training drills

- Not stating the problem clearly when help arrives.
- Not involving a consultant obstetrician and anaesthetist in the management of women with severe pre-eclampsia and eclampsia.
- Failure to adequately treat hypertension.
- Incorrect administration and labelling of magnesium sulphate.
- Failure to restrict fluids.
- Failure to stabilise the woman before delivery.
- Forgetting to perform basic resuscitation.

Introduction

Hypertensive disorders are the second most common cause of maternal death worldwide.[1] Between 2006 and 2008, 19 women in the UK died as a direct result of pre-eclampsia or eclampsia.[2] A further three women died as a result of acute fatty liver of pregnancy, which is thought to be related to the 'pre-eclampsia spectrum' of disease.

Unfortunately, the incidence of maternal death attributable to pre-eclampsia and eclampsia in the UK (currently 0.83/100 000 maternities) has not changed significantly over the last two decades[2] and the care of 20 of the 22 women who died in the last triennium was deemed to be substandard. In 14 cases this was classed as 'major', and these deaths could have been avoided with better care. Intracranial haemorrhage continues to be the single largest cause of death and indicates a failure of effective antihypertensive therapy.[2,3]

Severe hypertension (systolic blood pressure above 160 mmHg) must be treated to prevent maternal mortality and morbidity.[4]

Pre-eclampsia

Pre-eclampsia is a multisystem disorder of pregnancy characterised by new hypertension presenting after 20 weeks of gestation with significant proteinuria.[4] Pre-eclampsia is a disorder of the vascular endothelial function specific to pregnancy and is thought to arise in the placenta as a result of ischaemia.

Pre-eclampsia is one of the most common underlying causes of maternal and perinatal mortality (Box 6.1) and occurs in 3% of pregnancies.

Box 6.1 Maternal complications of pre-eclampsia

- Intracranial haemorrhage (leading cause of death from severe pre-eclamptic toxaemia in the UK)
- Placental abruption
- Eclampsia
- HELLP syndrome (characterised by haemolysis, elevated liver enzymes and low platelets)
- Disseminated intravascular coagulation
- Renal failure
- Pulmonary oedema
- Acute respiratory distress syndrome

Pre-eclampsia may also affect the fetus. Fetal complications are listed in Box 6.2.

Box 6.2 Fetal complications of pre-eclampsia

- Fetal growth restriction
- Oligohydramnios
- Hypoxia from placental insufficiency
- Placental abruption
- Premature delivery

Predisposing risk factors for pre-eclampsia are shown in Box 6.3.

Box 6.3 Predisposing risk factors for pre-eclampsia

- Nulliparity
- Hypertensive disease during a previous pregnancy
- Chronic hypertension
- Family history of pre-eclampsia
- Pre-existing diabetes
- Multiple pregnancy
- Obesity
- Extremes of maternal age
- Autoimmune disease (e.g. systemic lupus erythematosus, antiphospholipid syndrome)
- Renal disease
- Interval of 10 years or more since a previous pregnancy

Eclampsia

Eclampsia is defined as one or more convulsions in association with pre-eclampsia. Most women in the UK who have an eclamptic seizure will not have established hypertension and proteinuria prior to their first eclamptic seizure.[5] Forty-four percent of seizures occur postpartum, 38% antepartum and 18% intrapartum. The recurrence rate of seizures is 5–30%, even with treatment.

In the UK, the incidence of eclampsia has fallen to 2.7/10 000 maternities from 4.9/10 000 maternities in 1992.[6] There is a high rate of maternal complications associated with eclampsia, with at least one major morbidity in 10% of cases.[5] In the UK, the perinatal mortality associated with eclampsia is 10 times that of normal pregnancies.[5]

Presenting features

Eclampsia presents as generalised seizures, with jerking limb and head movements. The mother may become cyanosed, and tongue biting or urinary incontinence may also occur. Most seizures are single and self-limiting and usually resolve within 90 seconds. Eclampsia can be a very frightening experience for both family members and staff.

Management of eclampsia

The management of eclampsia involves basic life supportive measures as well as management of seizures. An outline for the initial management of eclampsia is shown in Figure 6.1. Management is described in more detail in the next section and is followed by details of the severe pre-eclampsia guidelines. Hypertension treatment guidelines are provided in the final section.

Call for help

Ring the emergency buzzer to summon help. This includes calling for a senior midwife, the most experienced obstetrician available, an anaesthetist and additional midwives and maternity care assistants to provide clinical support and document actions. Contact the consultant obstetrician and consultant anaesthetist.

■ Note the time the seizure occurred and its duration.

■ Note the time of the emergency call and time of arrival of staff.

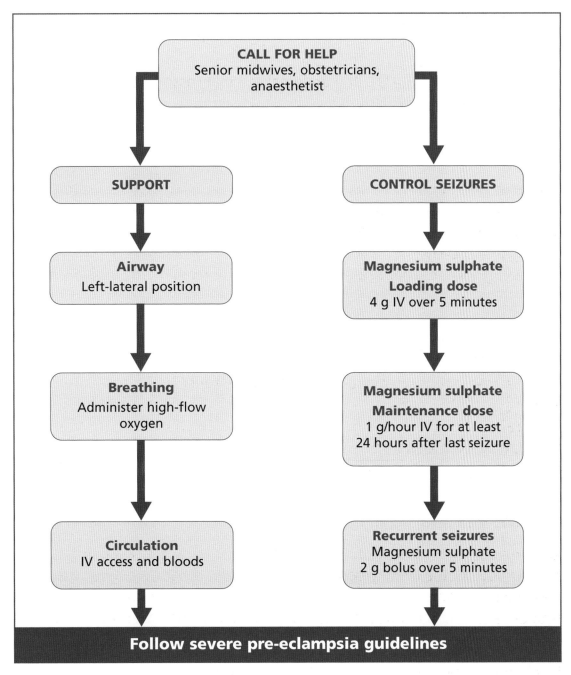

Figure 6.1 Outline of the initial management of eclampsia

Support: airway, breathing, circulation

Remember that most seizures are self-limiting. Remain calm. Monitor and maintain airway, breathing and circulation as your first priority. Move the mother into the left-lateral position and protect her from injury. Give high-flow facial oxygen by facemask with a reservoir bag. Do not attempt to restrain her during the seizure. Immediately following the eclamptic seizure, ensure the woman is maintained in the left-lateral position with an open airway.

Eclampsia box

Many units will have an emergency box containing a laminated treatment protocol as well as the emergency equipment and medication required for the immediate management of eclampsia (Figure 6.2).

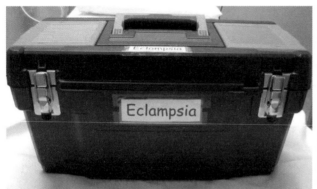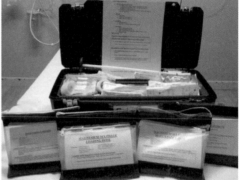

Figure 6.2 Eclampsia box with laminated treatment algorithm attached and showing contents

Control of seizures

Site a large-bore intravenous cannula and take bloods for full blood count, urea and electrolytes, liver function tests, clotting and group and save. Start treatment with magnesium sulphate.

> **Do not use diazepam, phenytoin or lytic cocktail as an alternative to magnesium sulphate in women with eclampsia.**

The results of the Collaborative Eclampsia trial demonstrated that women treated with magnesium sulphate have fewer recurrent seizures compared with women treated with diazepam or phenytoin.[7] Magnesium sulphate appears to act primarily by reducing cerebral vasospasm.[8] The intravenous route is preferable because intramuscular injections are painful and complicated by local abscess formation in 0.5% of cases.

The subsequent MAGPIE Trial demonstrated that magnesium sulphate can also prevent eclampsia (although the number of women needing treatment to prevent one woman having an eclamptic fit is high, particularly in the developed world).[9]

Magnesium sulphate emergency regimen

Loading dose: 4 g magnesium sulphate over 5 minutes

■ Draw up 8 ml of 50% magnesium sulphate solution (4 g) followed by 12 ml of 0.9% normal saline into a 20 ml syringe. This will give a total volume of 20 ml.

■ Give manually as an intravenous bolus over 5 minutes (4 ml/minute).

Maintenance dose: 1 g/hour

■ Draw up 20 ml of 50% magnesium sulphate solution (10 g) followed by 30 ml of 0.9% normal saline into a 50 ml syringe. This will give a total volume of 50 ml.

■ Place the syringe into a syringe driver and set the pump to run intravenously at 5 ml/hour.

■ Continue infusion for 24 hours following delivery or the last seizure, whichever is longest.

Recurrent seizures while on magnesium sulphate:

■ Seek immediate senior help.

■ Draw up 4 ml of 50% magnesium sulphate solution (2 g) followed by 6 ml of 0.9% saline into a 10 ml syringe. This will give a total volume of 10 ml.

■ Give as an intravenous bolus over 5 minutes (2 ml/minute).

■ If possible, take blood for magnesium levels prior to giving the bolus dose.

The maternal condition must be stabilised prior to making plans for birth (if antenatal).

Recurrent seizures may require treatment with diazepam or thiopentone/ propofol (if an anaesthetist is present). Consider other causes of seizures, such as intracranial haemorrhage, epilepsy, a space-occupying cerebral lesion or a cerebral vein thrombosis, and organise urgent imaging (CT, MRI or magnetic resonance venogram) as appropriate.

Magnesium sulphate is excreted in the urine by the kidneys. Magnesium toxicity is unlikely with this regimen and, if the woman has a normal urine output, the measurement of levels is not necessary. However, if the woman is oliguric (produces less than 100 ml urine over 4 hours) or has renal impairment, magnesium levels are more likely to become toxic and it is therefore advisable to administer the loading dose only. If the woman develops oliguria while receiving the maintenance dose of the magnesium sulphate infusion, this should be stopped and blood should be taken to measure the serum magnesium level. The therapeutic range for magnesium sulphate treatment is 2–4 mmol/l.

At toxic levels, there is a loss of deep tendon reflexes followed by respiratory depression, respiratory arrest and, ultimately, cardiac arrest. If maternal collapse occurs, follow the emergency protocol in Box 6.4. If toxicity is suspected, immediately stop the magnesium sulphate infusion and take blood for magnesium levels.

Box 6.4 Magnesium sulphate emergency protocol

CARDIOPULMONARY ARREST ON MAGNESIUM SULPHATE

- Stop magnesium sulphate infusion
- Start basic life support
- Give 1 g calcium gluconate IV (10 ml of 10% solution)
- Intubate early and ventilate until respiration resumes

Documentation

All personnel present at the emergency and all actions and treatment administered should be recorded as contemporaneously as possible. Figure 6.3 gives an example of an eclampsia documentation pro forma that may be used.

PROMPT
Making Childbirth Safer, Together

ECLAMPSIA PRO FORMA

DATE: .... TIME OF ECLAMPTIC FIT: .... DURATION OF ECLAMPTIC FIT: ....

PERSONS PRESENT AT ONSET OF ECLAMPTIC FIT...

....

EMERGENCY BELL ACTIVATED   YES / NO   TIME.....................

If emergency bell not activated, please give reason...

	NAME	ALREADY PRESENT (✓)	TIME INFORMED	TIME ARRIVED
EXPERIENCED OBSTETRICIAN				
MIDWIFE COORDINATOR				
ANAESTHETIST				
JUNIOR OBSTETRICIAN				
HCA				
OTHER PERSONS ASSISTING				

CONSLTANT OBSTETRICIAN INFORMED   YES / NO   Name...

If no, give reason...

Time attended (if attended)..

TREATMENT

LEFT LATERAL POSITION   YES / NO   TIME..................... If no, other position.......................................

HIGH FLOW O_2 YES / NO   TIME..................... If no, give reason.......................................

IV ACCESS   YES / NO   TIME..................... If no, give reason.......................................

BLOODS – GROUP + SAVE   YES / NO   TIME..................... If no, give reason.......................................

FBC, CLOTTING, U+E's, LFT's

URATE

MAGNESIUM SULPHATE INFUSION (see laminated regimen for dosages)	TIME COMMENCED
LOADING DOSE	
MAINTENANCE DOSE	

INITIAL POST ECLAMPTIC FIT OBSERVATIONS   TIME..................

RESP RATE............ PULSE RATE............... BP...........mm/Hg   02 sats...............% TEMP...................^{0}C

URINARY CATHETER INSERTED   YES / NO   TIME............. If no, give reason..

(Commence High Dependency Chart)

HYPERTENSIVE TREATMENT ADMINISTERED   YES/NO   TIME...................................

If yes, please document medication given and dosage...

....

Please complete AIMS form and attach copy of this pro forma – Thank you.

Figure 6.3 Example of eclampsia documentation pro forma

Severe pre-eclampsia management guidelines

Severe pre-eclampsia has been defined as:[4]

■ Severe hypertension (BP ≥ 160/110 mmHg) and proteinuria (urinary protein:creatinine ratio > 30 mg/mmol or 24-hour urine collection result shows > 300 mg protein)

  or

■ Mild or moderate hypertension (BP 140/90–159/109 mmHg) and proteinuria with at least one of the following:

☐ severe headache

☐ problems with vision such as blurring or flashing

☐ severe pain just below ribs or vomiting

☐ papilloedema

☐ signs of clonus (≥ 3 beats)

☐ liver tenderness

☐ HELLP syndrome

☐ platelet count falling to < 100 x 10^9/litre

☐ abnormal liver enzymes (ALT or AST rises to > 70 i.u./litre).

Note: Clinical discretion should be used to include women who present with atypical symptoms.[10]

Details of the management principles are outlined in Figure 6.4. These principles are discussed in more detail in the following section.

Management principles

The management of severe pre-eclampsia and eclampsia requires the initiation of complex treatment plans.[11] Local guidelines (based on current national guidance) should be available.

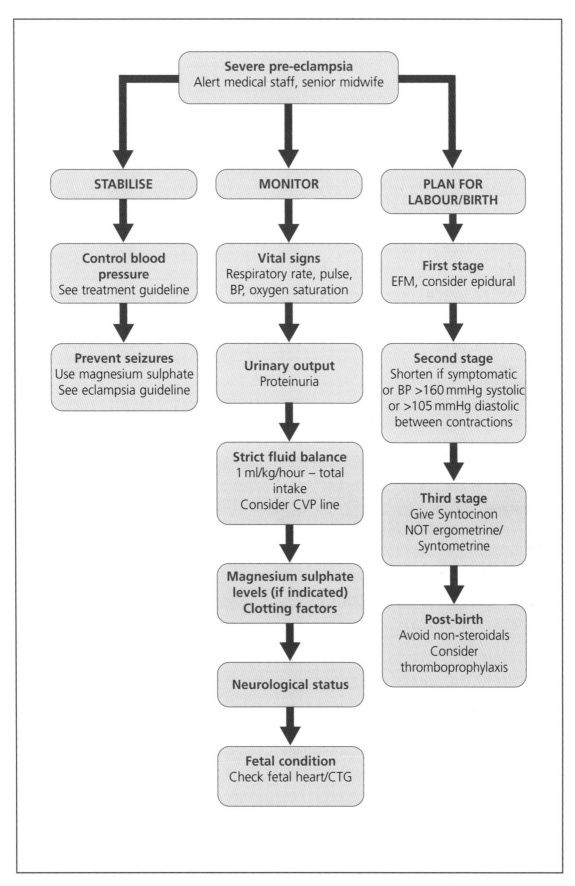

Figure 6.4 Outline of the management of severe pre-eclampsia

1. Stabilise

Effective and timely antihypertensive treatment is vital.[2,3]

Control of hypertension

In the latest triennial report on maternal deaths, the single major failing in critical care in deaths of women with eclampsia and pre-eclampsia was inadequate treatment of systolic hypertension, resulting in intracranial haemorrhage.[2] The exact mechanisms that link hypertension with intracranial haemorrhage are still unclear, but systolic hypertension poses the greatest risk. In addition, mean arterial pressure measurements may not always impart the real threat of a very high systolic blood pressure. The 2011 CMACE report suggests that, based on the evidence available, a systolic pressure of 160 mmHg or more requires urgent and effective antihypertensive treatment.[2] The report also identifies that pre-eclampsia can rapidly worsen, and in some circumstances treatment at less than 160 mmHg may be advisable (see Figure 6.5 for severe hypertension treatment flow chart). The NICE guideline recommends a target systolic pressure of below 150 mmHg.[4]

> **The 2011 CMACE report identified intracranial haemorrhage as the single largest cause of death from pre-eclampsia in the UK. A failure to administer effective antihypertensive therapy was implicated in most cases. Systolic hypertension poses the greatest risk and high pressures (>160 mmHg) should be treated as a medical emergency.[2]**

Any prescribed antihypertensive medication should be continued in labour and at caesarean section (usually labetalol and/or nifedipine). Anaesthetists and obstetricians should also be aware of the hypertensive effects of laryngoscopy and intubation when administering a general anaesthetic and control hypertension prior to intubation.[3]

Automated blood pressure recording devices can seriously underestimate blood pressure in pre-eclampsia. Blood pressure values should be compared at the beginning of treatment with those obtained by a manual device and an appropriately sized cuff should be used.[11] Consideration should be given to the use of an arterial line for difficult cases.

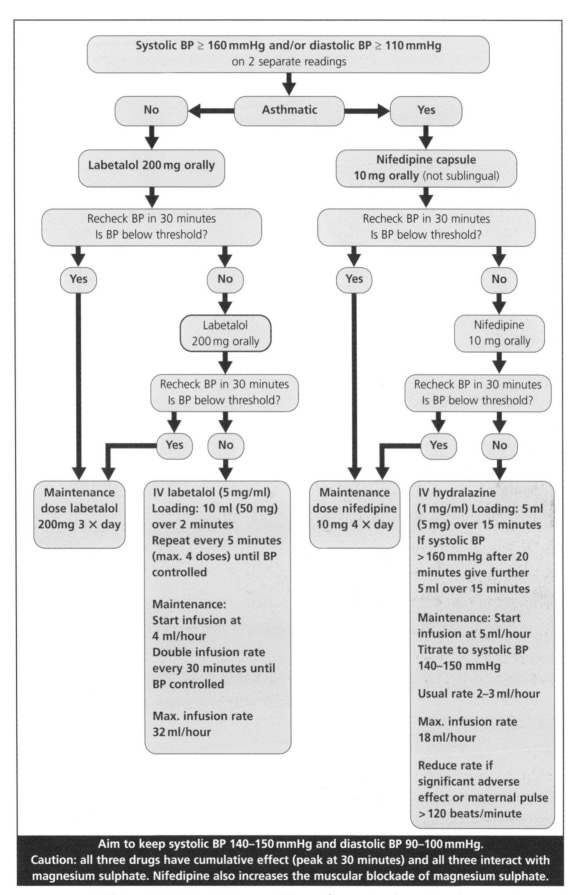

Figure 6.5 Treatment guidelines for severe hypertension

Prevent seizures

Consider giving intravenous magnesium sulphate to women with severe pre-eclampsia if birth is planned within 24 hours, especially if the woman is 30 weeks gestation or less, due to the added benefits of neuroprotection in the pre-term infant (RCOG Scientific Impact Paper No. 29, August 2011). Magnesium sulphate should be administered as per the eclampsia regimen; that is, a loading bolus dose followed by a maintenance infusion.

2. Monitor

A woman's condition can deteriorate rapidly. Vigilant observation and assessment is required and should be recorded on an obstetric high-dependency chart.

- Respiratory rate, pulse and blood pressure: every 15 minutes until stabilised, then every 30 minutes.
- Hourly urine output: Foley's catheter with urometer.
- Hourly oxygen saturations.
- Routine blood samples 12–24-hourly: FBC, clotting screen, U&Es, LFTs.

Additional observations and investigation for mothers receiving magnesium sulphate:

- Continuously monitor oxygen saturation.
- Hourly respiratory rate.
- Hourly deep tendon reflexes.
- If loss of reflexes, stop infusion and check magnesium levels:
  - ☐ If level less than 4 mmol/l or reflexes return, recommence infusion at 0.5 g/hour.
- If oliguric (less than 100 ml urine in 4 hours), magnesium levels should be taken.

Strict fluid balance

Close monitoring of fluid intake and urinary output is essential. Previous Confidential Enquiries have highlighted the risk of fluid overload causing pulmonary oedema in women with severe pre-eclampsia.

The maximum fluid intake (a combination of intravenous and oral intake) should be 1 ml/kg/hour. This is often approximated to 80 ml/hour. Beware of dilute drug administration and of excessive oxytocin which may inhibit urinary output.

All women with severe pre-eclampsia should have an indwelling urinary catheter, with a urometer for hourly urine measurement. All fluid input and output should be clearly documented on a high-dependency chart.

The aim is to 'run dry', as women die from fluid overload but rarely from renal failure. The intravenous fluid of choice (if required) for most cases will be Hartmann's solution (compound sodium lactate) or blood replacement if necessary.

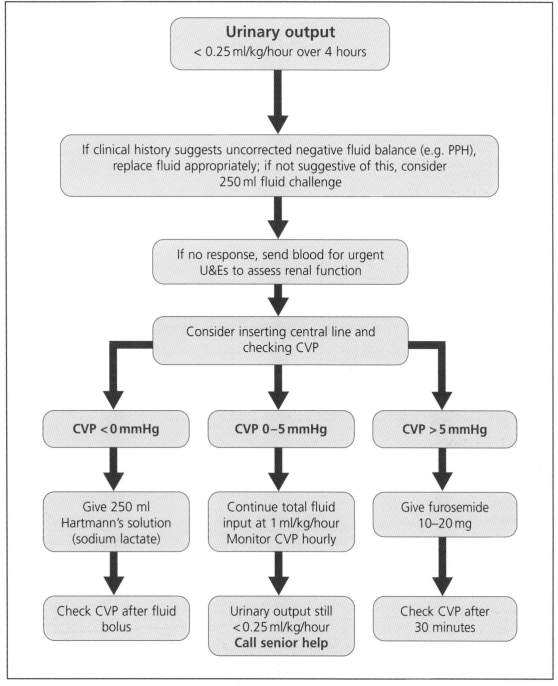

Figure 6.6 Fluid balance in the mother with oliguric pre-eclampsia

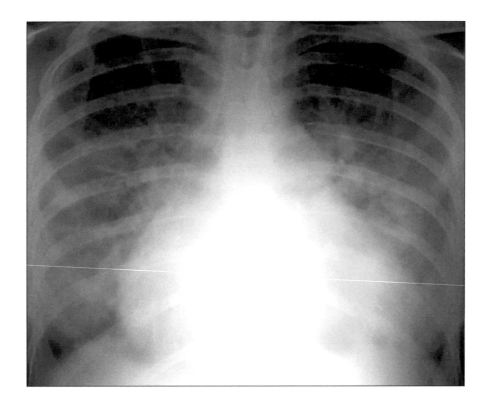

Figure 6.7 Chest X-ray showing the features of pulmonary oedema

Persistent oliguria (less than 100 ml of urine over 4 hours) requires careful management, as shown in Figure 6.6, and a central line should be considered. A central line may be helpful to aid fluid management when there are added complications such as a postpartum haemorrhage in a woman with severe pre-eclampsia. The aim is to maintain a central venous pressure between 0 mmHg and 5 mmHg. Great caution should be exercised with fluid treatment if the central venous pressure is greater than 5 mmHg.

Pulmonary oedema

Pulmonary oedema is defined as fluid accumulation in the lungs that leads to impaired gas exchange and may cause respiratory failure. Pulmonary oedema can occur secondary to pre-eclampsia because of hypoalbuminaemia, increased capillary permeability and a high hydrostatic pressure (hypertension). Thankfully, in the UK, pulmonary oedema is now a rare complication of pre-eclampsia as it has been recognised that it is essential to restrict fluids ('run the patient dry') and maintain an accurate fluid balance. Figure 6.7 shows an X-ray of the typical features of pulmonary oedema; however, clinical signs are usually sufficient to make the diagnosis (Box 6.5).

Box 6.5 Clinical signs and symptoms of pulmonary oedema

Symptoms of pulmonary oedema	Signs of pulmonary oedema
Shortness of breath	Tachypnoea
Unable to lie flat	Crepitations at lung bases
	Decreasing oxygen saturations
	Positive fluid balance
	Tachycardia
	Frothy sputum

The immediate management of pulmonary oedema is shown in Figure 6.8.

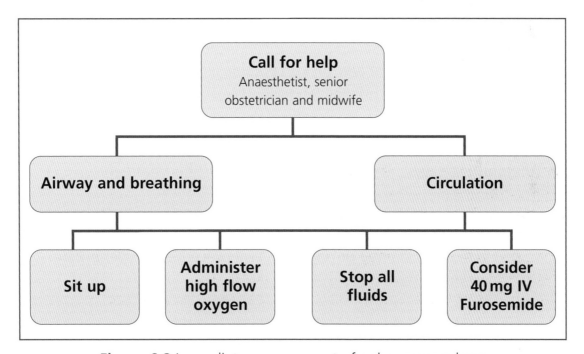

Figure 6.8 Immediate management of pulmonary oedema

Clotting abnormalities

Disseminated intravascular coagulation (DIC) is a potential complication of severe pre-eclampsia. Check activated partial thromboplastin time (APTT), prothrombin time and fibrinogen if platelet levels are less than 100×10^9. In addition, observe for clinical evidence of undue bleeding/bruises. If any of the investigations are abnormal, consider treatment with platelets and fresh frozen plasma (FFP) and liaise with the on-call clinical haematologist (more information can be found in **Module 2**).

3. Plan for labour/birth

Make plans for the birth of the baby once the mother's condition is stable. The choice of caesarean section or induction of labour should be made on an individual basis.

For the first stage of labour, close observation and the continuous attendance of an experienced midwife are required.

- Use continuous electronic fetal monitoring: there is increased risk of fetal hypoxia and placental abruption.
- Consider the use of epidural anaesthesia (pain tends to increase blood pressure). Do not preload women with IV fluids prior to epidural or spinal.[4]
- During labour measure BP every 15 minutes in women with severe hypertension or hourly in women with mild or moderate hypertension.

It is safe for the mother to have a normal active second stage of labour provided that she does not have a severe headache or visual disturbances and that her blood pressure is within acceptable limits (as per NICE guidance). Consider operative vaginal birth if:

- the mother complains of severe headache or visual disturbances
- the blood pressure is uncontrolled (greater than 160 mmHg systolic or 105 mmHg diastolic, between contractions) despite treatment.

The third stage of labour should be managed with 10 units of Syntocinon® (Alliance) IM (or slowly IV). Syntometrine and ergometrine should not be given to women with pre-eclampsia or eclampsia as it exacerbates hypertension.

Post-birth care

The mother will require continuous care after birth. This may be for several hours or several days, depending on the circumstances. Remember that most eclamptic seizures occur in the postnatal period and pre-eclampsia can worsen several days after birth. If symptoms arise, monitor and investigate. Women may require transfer back to the labour ward for clinical monitoring.

Ensure adequate analgesia but note that non-steroidal anti-inflammatory drugs such as diclofenac must not be given, as they can precipitate renal failure.

Consider the need for thromboprophylaxis as severe pre-eclampsia is a risk factor for thromboembolism. Apply thromboembolic deterrent stockings as soon as possible. Commence low-molecular-weight heparin post-birth provided that the mother's platelet count is greater than 100×10^9/litre.

Transfer to intensive therapy unit or high-dependency care

Previous Confidential Enquiries[10] and NICE[4] have highlighted that units should have documented procedures for the transfer of a mother to an intensive therapy unit.

Women should be treated in the appropriate setting[4] (Table 6.1).

Table 6.1 Treatment settings

Setting	Indication
Level 3 care: intensive therapy unit	Severe pre-eclampsia requiring ventilation
Level 2 care: high-dependency unit	Step down from level 3 or severe pre-eclamptic toxaemia with: ■ eclampsia ■ HELLP syndrome ■ haemorrhage ■ hyperkalaemia ■ severe oliguria ■ coagulation support ■ IV antihypertensive treatment ■ initial stabilisation of severe hypertension ■ evidence of cardiac failure ■ abnormal neurology
Level 1 care: ward patient needing critical care team input	■ Pre-eclampsia with mild or moderate hypertension ■ Continuing conservative antenatal management of severe preterm hypertension ■ Step-down treatment after the birth

References

1. Khan KS, Wojdyla D, Say L, Gülmezoglu AM, Van Look PF. WHO analysis of causes of maternal death: a systematic review. *Lancet* 2006;367:1066–74.

2. Centre for Maternal and Child Enquiries. Saving Mothers' Lives: reviewing maternal deaths to make motherhood safer: 2006–2008. The Eighth Report on Confidential Enquiries into Maternal Deaths in the United Kingdom. *BJOG* 2011;118 Suppl 1:1–203.

3. Lewis G (editor). *The Confidential Enquiry into Maternal and Child Health (CEMACH). Saving Mothers' Lives: Reviewing Maternal Deaths to Make Motherhood Safer 2003–2005. The Seventh Report on Confidential Enquiries into Maternal Deaths in the United Kingdom.* London: CEMACH; 2007.

4. National Collaborating Centre for Women's and Children's Health. *Hypertension in pregnancy: the management of hypertensive disorders during pregnancy.* NICE Clinical Guideline. London: Royal College of Obstetricians and Gynaecologists; 2011.

5. Knight M; UKOSS. Eclampsia in the United Kingdom 2005. *BJOG* 2007;114:1072–8.

6. Douglas KA, Redman CW. Eclampsia in the United Kingdom. *BMJ* 1994;309:1395–400.

7. Which anticonvulsant for women with eclampsia? Evidence from the Collaborative Eclampsia Trial. *Lancet* 1995;345:1455–63.

8. Naidu S, Payne AJ, Moodley J, Hoffmann M, Gouws E. Randomised study assessing the effect of phenytoin and magnesium sulphate on maternal cerebral circulation in eclampsia using transcranial Doppler ultrasound. *Br J Obstet Gynaecol* 1996;103:111–6.

9. Altman D, Carroli G, Duley L, Farrell B, Moodley J, Neilson J, et al.; Magpie Trial Collaboration Group. Do women with pre-eclampsia, and their babies, benefit from magnesium sulphate? The Magpie Trial: a randomised placebo-controlled trial. *Lancet* 2002;359:1877–90.

10. Lewis G (editor). The Confidential Enquiry into Maternal and Child Health (CEMACH). *Why Mothers Die 2000–2002. The Sixth Report on Confidential Enquiries into Maternal Deaths in the United Kingdom.* London: RCOG Press; 2004.

11. Royal College of Obstetricians and Gynaecologists. *The management of severe pre-eclampsia/eclampsia.* Green-top Guideline No. 10A. London: RCOG; 2006.

Module 7
Maternal sepsis

Key learning points

- Recognise severe maternal sepsis.
- Use of serum lactate to triage sepsis severity.
- Knowledge of the emergency management of septic shock.
- Need for early intravenous antibiotics and fluids.
- Importance of using modified obstetric early warning score charts.
- Importance of senior, multi-professional clinician involvement.
- Recall the potential complications of severe sepsis.

Common difficulties observed in training drills

- Not stating the problem.
- Failure to measure the patient's respiratory rate.
- Not plotting clinical observations on a modified obstetric early warning score (MOEWS) chart.
- Failure to recognise clinical features of sepsis.
- Delayed administration of antibiotics.
- Failure to treat sepsis with a fluid bolus.
- Failure to take microbiology cultures and serum lactate.
- Failure to summon appropriate senior support early.

Introduction

In the past, obstetricians and midwives were very aware of sepsis and its consequences. However, life-threatening sepsis has, until recently, been rare in the UK and many doctors and midwives will have never managed a case of severe maternal sepsis.

Before the introduction of antibiotics in the 1940s, genital tract sepsis was the leading cause of maternal death in the UK, accounting for over one-third of direct deaths occurring in pregnancy and childbirth. Since the introduction of antibiotics the number of maternal deaths attributable to sepsis has fallen dramatically.

However, recently there has been a concerning increase in maternal deaths attributable to sepsis, particularly those associated with group A streptococcal infection (GAS) (Table 7.1). During the 2006–08 triennium, sepsis was the leading cause of direct maternal deaths, accounting for 26 direct deaths, with a further three deaths classified as 'late direct'.[1] The majority of these deaths occurred in the postpartum period, and more than 50% followed a caesarean birth. However, seven women died from sepsis after vaginal birth, highlighting that even healthy women who have had a normal pregnancy and birth can rapidly become severely ill and die.

Table 7.1 Number and proportion of maternal deaths from sepsis in the UK

	1952–54	1985–87	2000–02	2003–05	2006–08
Rate/100 000 maternities	7.8	0.40	0.65	0.85	1.13
Number (all organisms)	–	9	13	21	29
Number (GAS)	–		3	8	13

Worldwide, sepsis remains a very important cause of maternal death: in 2005, over 80 000 women across the world died from pregnancy-related sepsis.[2]

What is sepsis?

Sepsis is the body's response to an infection following the invasion of the body by microorganisms, usually bacteria. The infection may be limited to a particular body region (e.g. chorioamnionitis) or may be widespread in the bloodstream, resulting in septicaemia. Sepsis is a medical emergency because it can result in an interruption of the supply of oxygen and nutrients to the tissues, including the vital organs such as the brain, heart, liver, kidneys, lungs and intestines, resulting in acidosis, organ failure and death.

Prevention of sepsis

The importance of hand washing, hygiene and antisepsis is well established in maternity care.

In the mid-19th century, Dr Semmelweis observed a marked increase in maternal mortality rates in patients under the care of doctors compared with those under the care of midwives in Vienna. He also noted that doctors coming straight from the autopsy room to the delivery room had a disagreeable smell on their hands despite washing with plain soap and water. He postulated that puerperal fever was caused by particles transmitted via the hands of the doctors. Semmelweis ordered a mandatory hand washing policy for doctors, requiring them to use a chlorinated solution before they examined women in labour. This intervention resulted in a dramatic fall in maternal mortality.[3]

Other techniques to reduce the incidence of maternal sepsis include barrier nursing, the use of antibiotic prophylaxis for preterm and prolonged rupture of membranes and the use of perioperative antibiotics for caesarean births, manual removal of placenta and anal sphincter tear repair.

Recognition of sepsis

The onset of life-threatening sepsis in pregnancy or the puerperium can be insidious or may show extremely rapid clinical deterioration, particularly when it is the result of streptococcal infection. In many of the sepsis-related maternal deaths reviewed by the Confidential Enquires in the UK, women had a short duration of illness and in some cases were moribund by the time they presented to hospital.

It is therefore essential that all staff, including community midwives, maternity care assistants, health visitors, emergency department staff and general practitioners, are aware of the signs and symptoms of sepsis. The potential severity of illness in women presenting with signs and symptoms of sepsis is often unrecognised or underestimated, resulting in delays in referral to hospital, delays in administration of appropriate antibiotic treatment and late involvement of senior medical staff.[4]

The 2006–08 Confidential Enquiry also stresses the importance of women themselves being informed of the risks, signs and symptoms of genital tract infection and the need for them to seek early advice if they are concerned.[1]

Signs and symptoms

Women with genital tract sepsis may present with abdominal pain, diarrhoea and vomiting. Some, but not all, will have a raised temperature. It can be very difficult to differentiate such symptoms from gastroenteritis, and therefore all pregnant or postnatal women presenting with such symptoms should be carefully examined. Women may also present antenatally with offensive vaginal discharge, or with increased and/or offensive lochia in the puerperium. Antenatally, the combination of abdominal pain and an abnormal or absent fetal heart rate may signify sepsis rather than placental abruption.

Many of the deaths in the most recent Confidential Enquiry were preceded by a sore throat or other upper respiratory tract infections.[1] All of the women who died from GAS either worked with, or had, young children.

Women may also present with a rash. The typical rash of streptococcus A (Figure 7.1) develops over 12–48 hours, first appearing as erythematous (red) patches on the chest and axillae which spread to the trunk and extremities. Typically, the rash consists of scarlet patches over generalised redness (a patchy sunburnt appearance). This rash will momentarily disappear with pressure, unlike the petechial rash typical of meningiococcal septicaemia.

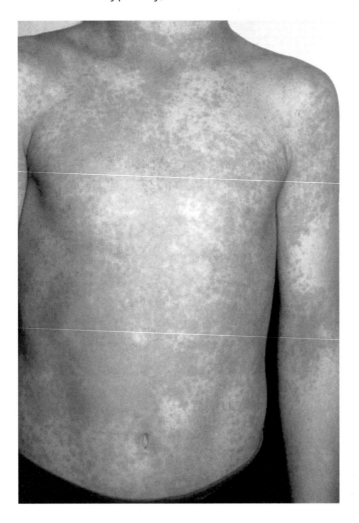

Figure 7.1 Streptococcus A rash

Women with severe sepsis may appear deceptively well. They may maintain their blood pressure and conceal serious illness for a prolonged period of time before sudden cardiovascular decompensation. It is therefore vital that basic clinical observations (heart rate, respiratory rate, blood pressure, temperature and, if available, oxygen saturations) are taken for every woman who presents with any of the symptoms in Box 7.1, or who simply 'just doesn't feel well'. The use of modified obstetric early warning score (MOEWS) charts to record physical observations is recommended, and should help in the early detection of women with sepsis.

Box 7.1 Signs and symptoms of genital tract sepsis

Symptoms	Signs
Fever	Rash (scarlet patches over generalised redness or petechial)
Diarrhoea	Tachycardia (heart rate > 100 bpm)
Vomiting	Tachypnoea/raised respiratory rate (respiratory rate > 24)
Abdominal pain	Pyrexia (> 38°C) or hypopyrexia (< 35°C)
Sore throat	
Upper respiratory tract infection	Hypotension (systolic blood pressure < 80 mmHg)
Vaginal discharge	Low oxygen saturations (< 95% on air)
Wound infection	Poor peripheral perfusion (capillary refill > 2 seconds)
	Pallor
	Clamminess
	Confusion
	Mottled skin
	Low urine output (< 0.5 ml/kg/hour)

Risk factors

Many women who present with sepsis will have no risk factors. Risk factors for sepsis are listed in Box 7.2 and potential causes of sepsis are listed in Box 7.3. In a postpartum woman with possible sepsis, any history of ragged membranes or possible incomplete delivery of the placenta should be sought, and the woman examined for the presence of uterine tenderness or enlargement.

Box 7.2 Risk factors for maternal sepsis

- Retained products of conception (following miscarriage, termination of pregnancy or delivery)
- Caesarean birth (an emergency caesarean birth carries a greater risk than an elective or planned procedure)
- Prolonged ruptured membranes
- Premature labour
- Wound haematoma
- Following an invasive intrauterine procedure (e.g. amniocentesis, chorionic villus sampling)
- Cervical suture
- Obesity
- Impaired immunity (e.g. immunosuppressants, high-dose steroids, HIV infection)
- Diabetes mellitus
- Working with, or having, young children

Box 7.3 Potential pregnancy- and non-pregnancy-related causes of maternal sepsis

Pregnancy related	Non-pregnancy related
Chorioamnionitis (following retained products of conception, prolonged ruptured membranes, caesarean birth, invasive procedures)	Appendicitis (may present atypically in pregnancy)
	Pyelonephritis (more common in pregnancy)
Postoperative (caesarean birth, cervical suture, haematoma, amniocentesis)	Cholecystitis
	Bowel perforation (more common with inflammatory bowel disease)
Breast abscess	Meningitis
	Pneumonia
	Cellulitis

Management

The Surviving Sepsis Campaign is a global initiative aimed at reducing mortality from sepsis by building awareness, improving diagnosis, increasing the use of appropriate treatment, educating healthcare professionals and developing guidelines for care. More information about the Surviving Sepsis Campaign can be found at www.survivingsepsis.org.[5]

Maternal sepsis can be challenging to manage, but better training, a structured approach, earlier recognition and good care in both community and hospital settings may help to save lives. Prompt investigation and treatment, particularly immediate intravenous antibiotic treatment, intravenous fluids and early involvement of senior clinical staff, is crucial.

The management of severe maternal sepsis requires the rapid initiation of multiple overlapping actions. The exact sequence will be dictated by the needs of the individual mother and the resources available. An outline for the initial management of sepsis is shown in Figure 7.2. Management is described in more detail in the next section.

Call for help

Early involvement of senior midwives, obstetricians, anaesthetists and critical care consultants is crucial.

Support: airway, breathing, circulation

Monitor and maintain airway, breathing and circulation as your first priority. If the woman has collapsed, check that her airway is patent and that she is breathing. Give high-flow oxygen by facemask with a reservoir bag and ensure the woman is maintained in the left-lateral postion. Secure intravenous access as soon as possible.

Prompt early intravenous antibiotic treatment

Immediate high-dose broad-spectrum intravenous antibiotic therapy (e.g. 1.5 g cefuroxime and 500 mg metronidazole), in accordance with local prescribing guidelines and known patient allergies, should be commenced as soon as possible.[4] Antibiotic administration should not be delayed to await results of microbiological testing. If possible, blood cultures should be taken prior to the administration of antibiotics but, again, the commencement of antibiotic treatment should not be delayed.

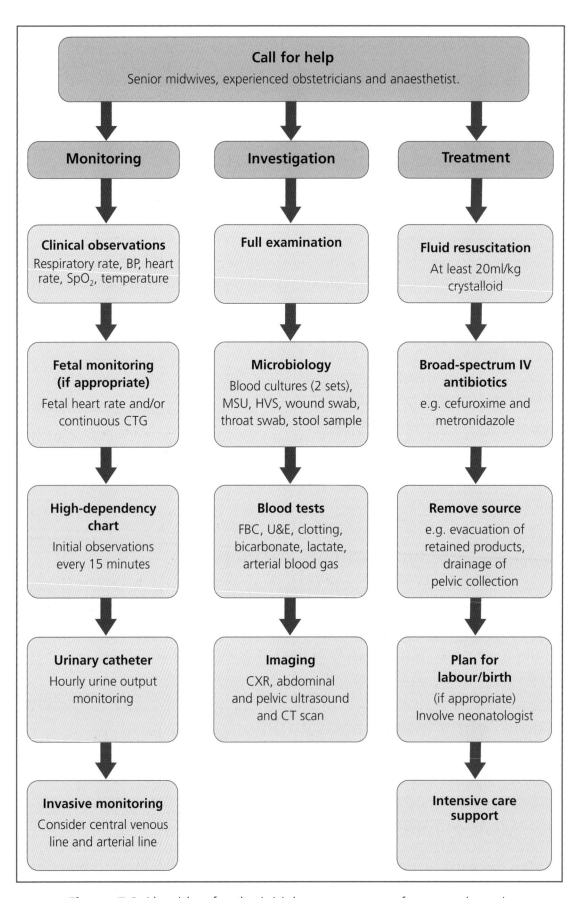

Figure 7.2 Algorithm for the initial management of maternal sepsis

A microbiologist should be contacted early for advice. If the woman is already extremely ill, deteriorates or does not improve within 24 hours of treatment, additional or alternative intravenous antibiotics such as gentamicin and clindamycin or piperacillin/tazobactam (Tazocin®; Wyeth) should be used.

Fluid resuscitation

Hypotension and/or an elevated serum lactate level (> 4 mmol/l) should be treated with intravenous fluid. Women should be given an initial minimum fluid challenge of 20 ml/kg of intravenous crystalloid.[4] This means a 75 kg patient with sepsis should be given at least 1500 ml of intravenous crystalloid. If there is no improvement in the hypotension and/or the serum lactate level following the fluid bolus, the patient should be transferred to intensive care where vasopressors can be administered to maintain the mean arterial pressure above 65 mmHg.

Full clinical examination

A full clinical examination should be performed with the aim of identifying the cause of the sepsis. This should be a top-to-toe examination including a vaginal examination to exclude retained tampons or swabs.

Monitor

Women with maternal sepsis can deteriorate rapidly. Vigilance in observation and assessment is required and vital signs should be recorded on a MOEWS chart. This may aid the early detection of a deteriorating patient.

- Respiratory rate, pulse, blood pressure and oxygen saturations: every 15 minutes until stabilised, then every 30 minutes.
- At least 4-hourly temperature.
- Hourly urine output: Foley catheter with urometer.
- Blood samples 4–12-hourly depending on clinical condition: full blood count, clotting screen, urea and electrolytes, liver function tests, bicarbonate and lactate.

Microbiology testing

Swabs or cultures should be taken from all potential sources of sepsis. Samples should be sent urgently to the microbiology laboratory, where immediate microscopy should be performed on appropriate samples. The results of microbiology testing should be promptly followed up and antibiotic treatment altered accordingly. Samples should include:

■ blood cultures (from at least two separate sites and from all intravenous cannulas that have been in place for longer than 48 hours)

■ vaginal swabs

■ urine culture

■ wound swabs

■ throat swab

■ stool sample

■ sputum sample

■ placental swabs (if immediately postpartum).

The most common pathogen associated with death from genital tract sepsis in the UK is group A beta-haemolytic streptococcus, also known as puerperal sepsis, childbed fever or Strep A. Other pathogens which commonly cause genital tract sepsis include *Escherichia coli*, group B beta-haemolytic streptococcus, *Staphylococcus aureus*, coagulase-negative staphylococcus, pseudomonas and mixed anaerobes/bacteroides species. Many women with genital tract sepsis will have a mixed infection with two or more organisms.

Blood tests

Full blood count

The white blood cell count (WBC) is commonly raised (greater than 14) with a high neutrophil count in sepsis. However, the WBC may also be low (less than 4), indicating severe sepsis. The platelet count may be low or raised.

Renal and liver function

Acute tubular necrosis may develop, which can lead to renal failure with raised urea, creatinine and potassium levels. The proinflammatory state of sepsis can also lead to hyperbilirubinaemia and jaundice.

Clotting studies

Disseminated intravascular coagulation (DIC) is a potential complication of severe sepsis. The activated partial thromboplastin time (APTT), prothrombin time and fibrinogen should be checked. In addition, observe for clinical evidence of undue bleeding/bruising. If any of the investigations are abnormal, consider treatment with platelets, fresh frozen plasma (FFP) and/or cryopreciptate and liaise with the on-call clinical haematologist.

Serum lactate

Patients with severe sepsis or septic shock typically have a high serum lactate which may be secondary to anaerobic metabolism attributable to poor tissue perfusion. A lactate level greater than 4 mmol/l indicates a poor prognosis.[6] Obtaining a lactate level is essential for identifying tissue hypoperfusion in patients who are not yet hypotensive but who are at risk of septic shock.

An arterial blood gas analyser located on the labour ward or in the neonatal intensive care unit will often be able to measure a serum lactate level.

Because of the high risk of septic shock, the Surviving Sepsis Campaign recommends that any patient with an elevated serum lactate level (>4 mmol/l) is given an initial minimum of 20 ml/kg of crystalloid fluid, regardless of their blood pressure. If there is no improvement in the serum lactate level following the fluid bolus, the patient should be transferred to intensive care for inotropic support.

Arterial blood gas

An arterial blood gas is a very useful investigation in any patient who is unwell.

It is likely to show metabolic acidosis (arterial pH < 7.35) owing to the production of lactate, as mentioned above. Respiratory compensation can occur in the form of hyperventilation leading to a low $PaCO_2$, but this will never completely correct the low pH. Serum bicarbonate is usually low (normal value 24–33 mmol/l) as bicarbonate is consumed in buffering hydrogen ions and serum lactate increases. As shock progresses, metabolic acidosis worsens, compensatory mechanisms are exhausted and blood pH decreases further (< 7.2). Early respiratory failure can lead to hypoxia with PaO_2 < 8 kPa.

Remove the source of maternal sepsis

If possible, the source of sepsis should be removed. Delivery should be expedited if there are signs of chorioamnionitis. Severe maternal infection can also affect the fetus and therefore neonatal advice should be sought.

Any retained products of conception should be removed as soon as the maternal condition is stable. A laparotomy and sometimes hysterectomy may be necessary.

Imaging

Imaging may help to identify the source of the sepsis:

- abdominal ultrasound for retained products of conception or abdominal collection
- chest X-ray
- computed tomography of the chest, abdomen and pelvis.

Prophylactic treatment

Women with sepsis are at increased risk of venous thromboembolism. Deep venous thrombosis prophylaxis with low-molecular-weight heparin and/or the use of compression stockings should be considered.

Multi-professional approach

Early advice should be sought from other specialists, such as anaesthetists, intensive care specialists, haematologists and microbiologists as well as obstetricians. Critically ill patients should be cared for in a high-dependency or intensive care unit.

> **There is a need to raise both maternal and professional awareness regarding antenatal, intrapartum and puerperal sepsis. Local guidelines and protocols should be available to all maternity unit and emergency department staff, as well as general practitioners and community midwives, so that maternal sepsis can be promptly recognised and managed.[1]**

References

1. Centre for Maternal and Child Enquiries. *CMACE Emergent Theme Briefing #1: Genital Tract Sepsis. Saving Mothers' Lives 2006–08: Briefing on genital tract sepsis.* London: CMACE; 2010.

2. Betrán AP, Wojdyla D, Posner SF, Gülmezoglu AM. National estimates for maternal mortality: an analysis based on the WHO systematic review of maternal mortality and morbidity. *BMC Public Health* 2005;5:131.

3. Sumbul M, Parapia LA. Handwashing and hygiene: lessons from history. *J R Coll Physicians Edinb* 2008;38:379.

4. Lewis G (editor). The Confidential Enquiry into Maternal and Child Health (CEMACH). *Saving Mothers' Lives: Reviewing Maternal Deaths to Make Motherhood Safer 2003–2005. The Seventh Report on Confidential Enquiries into Maternal Deaths in the United Kingdom.* London: CEMACH; 2007.

5. Surviving Sepsis Campaign; 2011 [http://www.survivingsepsis.org].

6. Weil MH, Afifi AA. Experimental and clinical studies on lactate and pyruvate as indicators of the severity of acute circulatory failure (shock). *Circulation* 1970;41:989–1001.

Module 8

Major obstetric haemorrhage

Key learning points

■ To understand the main risk factors for and causes of major obstetric haemorrhage.

■ To understand the importance of early recognition of obstetric haemorrhage.

■ To be familiar with the immediate management and specific treatment of major antepartum, intrapartum and postpartum haemorrhage.

■ To emphasise the importance of early adequate fluid resuscitation.

■ To communicate effectively with the woman and the multi-professional team.

■ Document details of management accurately, clearly and legibly.

Common difficulties observed in training drills

■ Delay in recognition of the severity of the problem until the woman becomes shocked.

■ Failure to promptly recognise concealed bleeding.

■ Not stating the problem clearly to all who attend the emergency.

■ Delay in commencing adequate fluid resuscitation.

■ Delay in recognising need to proceed to operative intervention.

- Uncertainty about how to access blood products rapidly.
- Injudicious use of misoprostol.

Introduction

Massive obstetric haemorrhage is the leading cause of maternal death worldwide, accounting for at least 50% of deaths in some series.[1]

In the UK, major obstetric haemorrhage complicates 3.7/1000 births,[2] with a maternal mortality of 3.9/million maternities.[3] Over 50% of the women who died had received 'major substandard care', implying that if care had been better these women would probably have survived.[3] In particular, there was a lack of early senior multi-professional involvement, a lack of close postoperative monitoring, failure to act on signs and symptoms and inadequate use and interpretation of modified obstetric early warning score (MOEWS) charts.

Definition of haemorrhage

Antepartum haemorrhage (APH) is defined as bleeding from the genital tract after the 24th week of pregnancy. It can occur at any time until the onset of labour.

Intrapartum haemorrhage is defined as bleeding from the genital tract at any time during labour until the completion of the second stage of labour.

Primary postpartum haemorrhage (PPH) is traditionally defined as a blood loss of 500 ml or more within the first 24 hours after delivery. However, most healthy women can cope with this amount of blood loss without problems. A major PPH is defined as a blood loss greater than 1000 ml.[4]

Secondary PPH is defined as a blood loss of 500 ml or more from 24 hours postpartum up until 12 weeks postpartum.[4]

Pathophysiology

The normal adult blood volume is approximately 70 ml/kg, which amounts to a total blood volume of about 5 litres. The healthy pregnant woman has a total blood volume of 6–7 litres in late pregnancy. This increased blood volume, in conjunction with increased levels of blood coagulation factors such as fibrinogen and clotting factors VII, VIII and X, provides physiological protection against haemorrhage.

Blood loss can be difficult to estimate and bleeding can be concealed within the uterus, broad ligament or uterine cavity. Normal blood loss (< 500 ml) at a vaginal birth or at a caesarean birth will not change the maternal pulse or blood pressure; however, more significant losses definitely will. Table 8.1 summarises the clinical features of shock in pregnancy related to the volume of blood loss.

Table 8.1 Clinical features of shock in pregnancy related to blood loss

Blood loss (ml)	Clinical features	Level of shock
500–1000	Normal blood pressure Tachycardia Palpitations, dizziness	Compensated
1000–1500	Hypotension systolic 90–80 mmHg Tachycardia Tachypnoea (21–30 breaths/minute) Pallor, sweating Weakness, faintness, thirst	Mild
1500–2000	Hypotension 80–60 mmHg Rapid, weak pulse > 110 beats/minute Tachypnoea (> 30 breaths/minute) Pallor, cold clammy skin Poor urinary output < 30 ml/hour Restlessness, anxiety, confusion	Moderate
2000–3000	Severe hypotension < 50 mmHg Pallor, cold clammy skin, peripheral cyanosis Air hunger Anuria Confusion or unconsciousness, collapse	Severe

Coagulopathies may develop as a consequence of severe blood loss. In disseminated intravascular coagulation (DIC), blood is exposed to excessive amounts of clotting factors including thromboplastin. Coagulation factors are consumed rapidly and the fibrinolytic system is activated, causing disruption to the control of coagulation balance and fibrinolysis. This may increasingly deteriorate until haemostasis is no longer possible.

Protocol for major obstetric haemorrhage

All maternity units should have an obstetric haemorrhage protocol for cases of major haemorrhage and the multi-professional team should update and rehearse this protocol regularly in conjunction with haematology and blood bank staff.[3,4]

Fluid resuscitation

Fluid resuscitation to restore the circulating volume is a priority in any major obstetric haemorrhage.

Fluid resuscitation and administration of blood products are key elements in the management of any major haemorrhage. It should be noted that maternal blood loss is notoriously difficult to quantify and often tends to be underestimated. Figure 8.1 may be used as an 'aide memoir' for estimating blood loss.

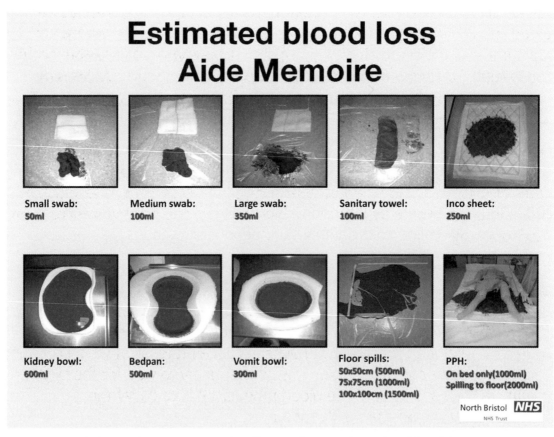

Figure 8.1 An example of a guide to estimating blood loss
(as per S Paterson-Brown model: Bose P, et al. *BJOG* 2006;113:919–24)

Immediate large intravenous access and fluid replacement

At least two large-bore (14G or 16G, 'grey or brown') intravenous cannulas should be sited. As the lines are established, blood should be taken for full blood count, clotting and cross-matching. Crystalloid solutions (e.g. Hartmann's solution or 0.9% saline) are the first-line choice for early fluid replacement. Warmed fluids should be infused as rapidly as possible until the systolic blood pressure has been restored.

Volume to be infused

Three litres of clear fluids (crystalloids and colloids) should be administered[5,6] and consideration should then be given to replacing blood by the most appropriate product (see below).

Give blood and blood products

In massive haemorrhage, the blood volume and oxygen-carrying capacity need to be restored. While careful consideration should always be given to the decision to transfuse, when there is major haemorrhage, compatible blood should be transfused as soon as possible (using a blood warmer or rapid infuser). It is preferable to give blood of the same group as the mother. However, if fully cross-matched blood is not available after three litres of clear intravenous fluids have been given, or if the bleeding is massive and unrelenting, transfuse with O-negative or type-specific blood.

Near-patient tests such as haemoglobin assessment with the HemoCue® (HemoCue AB, Ängelholm, Sweden) and thromboelastography are vital in cases of massive, rapid haemorrhage because there are often unavoidable delays in obtaining the results of full blood counts and clotting screens from the laboratory.

It should be remembered that transfusing a 'unit of blood' replaces red blood cells only, not clotting factors or platelets. Therefore, in massive haemorrhage, early consideration should be given to transfusing fresh frozen plasma (FFP), cryoprecipitate (which provides a more concentrated source of fibrinogen than FFP) and platelet concentrate, all of which contain vital components for coagulation. It is not necessary to wait for the clotting results before transfusing these blood products. It is vital that the haematologist is contacted early for advice.

The RCOG recommends that up to 1 litre of FFP and two packs of cryoprecipitate (10 units) can be given while the clotting results are awaited.

The aim is to keep the prothrombin time and activated partial thromboplastin time (APTT) to less than 1.5 × mean control. The dose of FFP is 12–15 ml/kg, which generally equates to giving 4 units of FFP for every 6 units of red blood cells.[4]

Cell salvage

Intraoperative cell salvage (the process whereby blood lost during an operation is collected, filtered and washed and transfused back into the patient) is commonly used in general surgery and significantly reduces the need for donor blood transfusion. This process is now increasingly used in obstetrics, especially for women who refuse blood or blood products, or where massive blood loss is anticipated (placenta percreta or accreta).[4]

With cell salvage, there is potential for maternal sensitisation in rhesus-negative women owing to contamination with fetal red cells; therefore, the standard dose of anti-D should be given and a Kleihauer test taken 1 hour after cell salvage has finished to determine whether further anti-D is required.[4] Care should also be taken to ensure the salvaged blood is not contaminated with amniotic fluid.

Antenatal risk assessment for haemorrhage

Anaemia

Anaemia magnifies the effects of obstetric haemorrhage because women who are anaemic are less able to tolerate blood loss. Important aspects of antenatal care include antenatal screening of haemoglobin levels and treatment of anaemia.

Haemorrhagic disorders

Mothers with inherited haemorrhagic disorders, such as haemophilia and von Willebrand's disease, are at an increased risk of haemorrhage and therefore require specialist care throughout pregnancy, with clear individualised plans for intrapartum and postpartum care documented in the woman's notes.

Pre-eclampsia complicated by HELLP syndrome (haemolysis, elevated liver enzymes, low platelets) may also make the mother vulnerable to bleeding.

Placenta praevia and accreta

Placenta praevia, particularly in mothers with a previous uterine scar, may be associated with uncontrollable uterine haemorrhage at delivery and caesarean hysterectomy may be necessary. Senior obstetricians and anaesthetists should both plan and perform the caesarean section. Consideration and planning for the use of cell salvage and interventional radiology are also recommended.

Women who decline blood products

Women who may decline blood products should be identified in the antenatal period. A clear plan for the management of potential haemorrhage should be documented in the maternal notes. This plan should identify specific blood products and treatments that would be acceptable to the woman (including cell salvage). The principles of the management of haemorrhage in these cases are to avoid delay, ensure senior assistance is summoned early and to have early recourse to use of pharmacological, radiological and surgical interventions.[3]

The use of modified obstetric early warning score (MOEWS) charts

It is important to be especially vigilant with women who are at risk of haemorrhage and to recognise signs and symptoms of bleeding as early as possible. CMACE highlights failure to pick up the signs and symptoms of intra-abdominal bleeding, particularly after caesarean section, and recommends the use of MOEWS charts (Figure 8.2) to address this problem.[3]

The use of the MOEWS chart should alert care-givers (including MCAs, who have an increasing role as part of the maternity team) to abnormal trends. However, 'trigger charts' are useful only if measurements are accurately plotted and action is taken appropriately after alerts.

Antepartum haemorrhage

APH complicates 2–5% of all pregnancies.[7] APH is often unpredictable, and the woman's condition may deteriorate rapidly before, during or after the onset of haemorrhage.

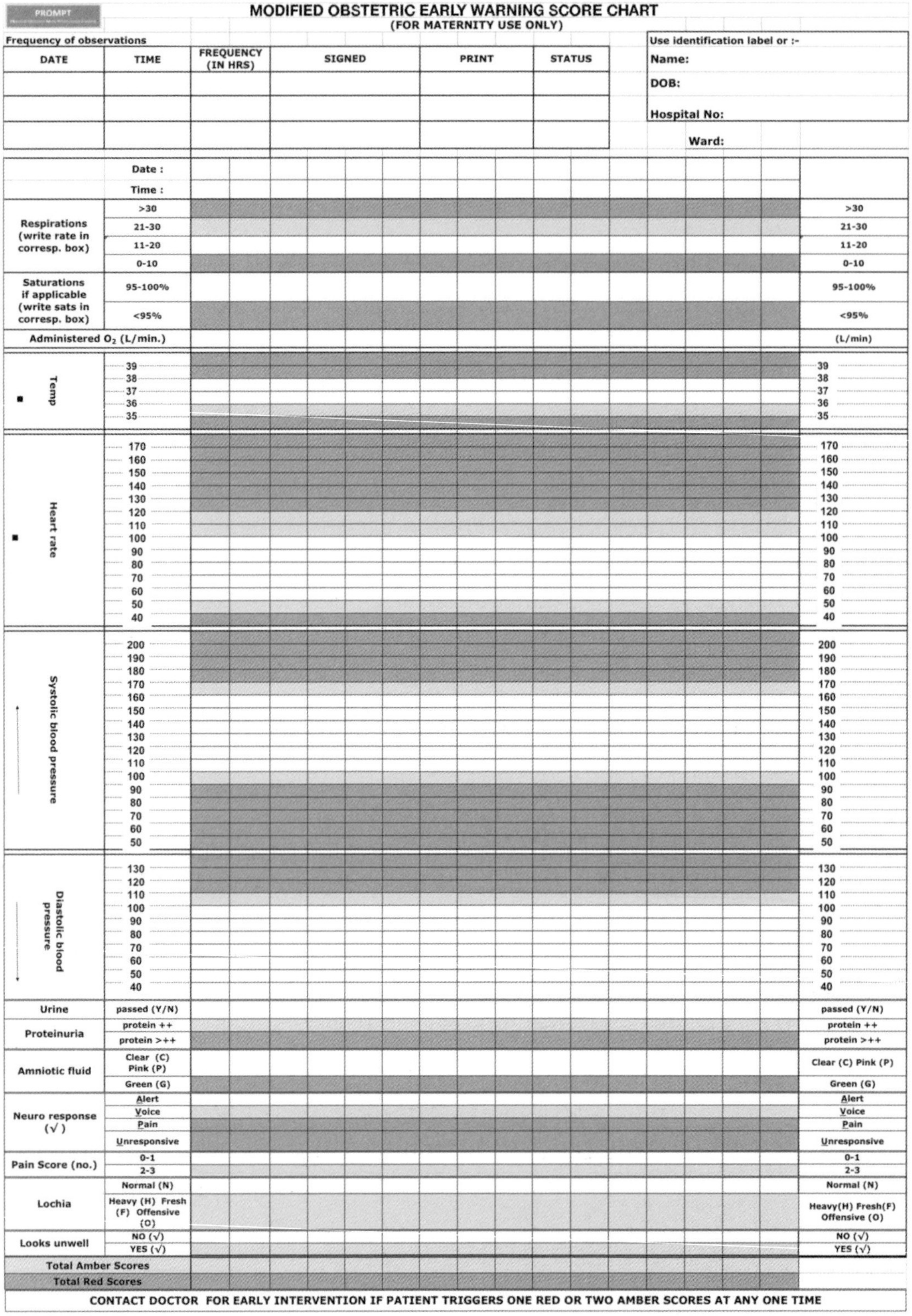

PROMPT

MODIFIED OBSTETRIC EARLY WARNING SCORE CHART
(FOR MATERNITY USE ONLY)

Frequency of observations

DATE	TIME	FREQUENCY (IN HRS)	SIGNED	PRINT	STATUS

Use identification label or :-
Name:
DOB:
Hospital No:
Ward:

	Date :		
	Time :		
Respirations (write rate in corresp. box)	>30		>30
	21-30		21-30
	11-20		11-20
	0-10		0-10
Saturations if applicable (write sats in corresp. box)	95-100%		95-100%
	<95%		<95%
Administered O_2 (L/min.)			(L/min)
▪ Temp	39		39
	38		38
	37		37
	36		36
	35		35
▪ Heart rate	170		170
	160		160
	150		150
	140		140
	130		130
	120		120
	110		110
	100		100
	90		90
	80		80
	70		70
	60		60
	50		50
	40		40
Systolic blood pressure	200		200
	190		190
	180		180
	170		170
	160		160
	150		150
	140		140
	130		130
	120		120
	110		110
	100		100
	90		90
	80		80
	70		70
	60		60
	50		50
Diastolic blood pressure	130		130
	120		120
	110		110
	100		100
	90		90
	80		80
	70		70
	60		60
	50		50
	40		40
Urine	passed (Y/N)		passed (Y/N)
Proteinuria	protein ++		protein ++
	protein >++		protein >++
Amniotic fluid	Clear (C) Pink (P)		Clear (C) Pink (P)
	Green (G)		Green (G)
Neuro response (√)	Alert		Alert
	Voice		Voice
	Pain		Pain
	Unresponsive		Unresponsive
Pain Score (no.)	0-1		0-1
	2-3		2-3
Lochia	Normal (N)		Normal (N)
	Heavy (H) Fresh (F) Offensive (O)		Heavy(H) Fresh(F) Offensive (O)
Looks unwell	NO (√)		NO (√)
	YES (√)		YES (√)
Total Amber Scores			
Total Red Scores			

CONTACT DOCTOR FOR EARLY INTERVENTION IF PATIENT TRIGGERS ONE RED OR TWO AMBER SCORES AT ANY ONE TIME

Figure 8.2 An example of a MOEWS chart and guidance for use

Causes of APH

The most common causes of minor APH are marginal placental bleeds, bleeding from a cervical ectropion or a blood-stained 'show'.

The most common causes of major APH are placental abruption and placenta praevia. Uterine rupture (secondary to the forces of labour, or abdominal trauma including road traffic accidents) can also lead to massive haemorrhage.

Ruptured vasa praevia may cause catastrophic APH for the fetus. Although ruptured vasa praevia is not associated with major maternal blood loss, it is an obstetric emergency owing to the rapid development of acute fetal anaemia.

Clinical presentation of major APH

A woman with an APH usually presents with obvious vaginal bleeding; however, bleeding may be concealed and therefore haemorrhage must be considered in any pregnant women with signs or symptoms of shock or a history of collapse.

Table 8.2 lists the presenting features and causes of APH.

Initial management of major APH

Major APH is a serious obstetric emergency. Blood loss can be torrential with rapid deterioration in the maternal and fetal condition. Remember that blood loss is often underestimated and may be concealed, especially in the case of uterine rupture or placental abruption.

The management of a major APH requires the prompt initiation of multiple simultaneous actions. Rapid assessment of fetal and maternal wellbeing is required. The initial management to stabilise the maternal condition will be the same regardless of the cause of bleeding. This should be followed by specific treatment measures dependent on the cause. The exact sequence will be dictated by the needs of the individual mother, the fetal condition and the resources available.

An outline of the initial management for a major APH is shown in Figure 8.3. This is discussed in more detail in the following section.

Table 8.2 Presenting features and causes of APH

Cause	Possible presenting features	Condition of uterus	Condition of fetus	Risk factors/ contributory factors
Placenta praevia	Painless vaginal bleeding High presenting part or transverse lie Shock	Non-tender and soft or irritable uterus	Dependent on amount of blood loss	Previous uterine surgery e.g. caesarean section Low-lying placenta on antenatal ultrasound
Placental abruption	Bleeding (may be concealed) Constant pain Shock Fetal compromise Pathological CTG	Tender, woody, hard uterus Irritable uterus	Dependent on blood loss and timing since abruption occurred	Previous abruption (up to 25% recurrence rate if two previous abruptions)[8] Pre-eclampsia Hypertension Fetal growth restriction Cocaine use Smoking Abdominal trauma Advanced maternal age Grand multiparity
Uterine rupture	Sudden onset of constant sharp pain Peritonism Abnormal/ pathological CTG Very high or unreachable presenting part Bleeding (may be concealed) Shock Haematuria	Contractions may cease	Likely to have abnormal/ pathological CTG Palpated ex utero	Previous uterine surgery (caesarean section/ myomectomy/corneal ectopic pregnancy) ≥ 4 parity Trauma Oxytocin infusion
Vasa praevia	Variable fresh PV blood loss after rupture of membranes Acute fetal compromise No maternal shock	Normal	Acute fetal compromise – sinusoidal / bradycardic CTG Fetal mortality 33–100%	Low-lying placenta Succenturiate lobe

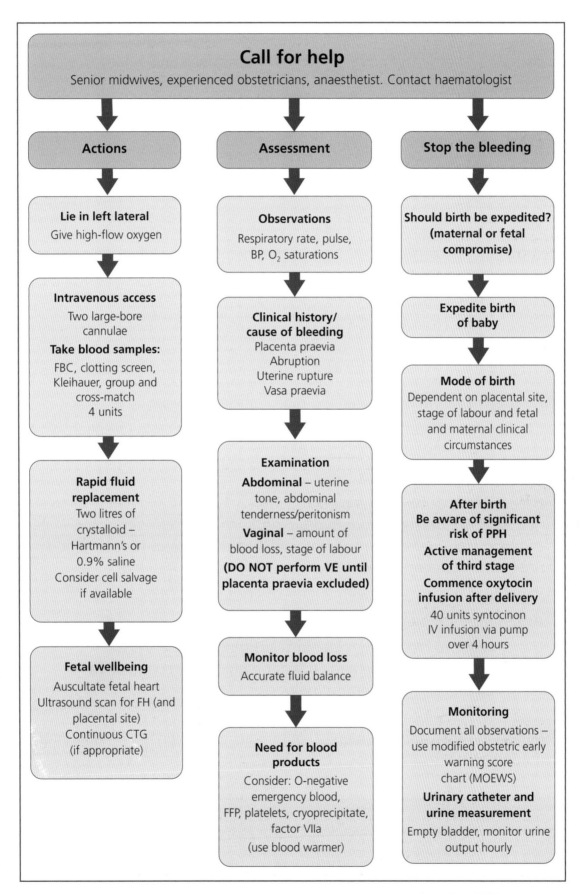

Figure 8.3 Algorithm for the initial management of major APH

CALL FOR HELP

Activate the emergency buzzer to summon assistance and emergency call for the appropriate personnel:

- senior midwife
- experienced obstetrician
- experienced anaesthetist
- experienced neonatologist
- additional support staff.

Alert the haematologist, blood bank technician, theatre staff and porter to be on standby as the major obstetric haemorrhage protocol may be activated and management of the woman in theatre may be required. The consultant obstetrician and anaesthetist should also be informed.

ACTIONS

- Lie the woman in left lateral and give high-flow oxygen.
- Clinical observations (pulse, blood pressure, capillary refill, respiratory rate and oxygen saturations).
- Site two large intravenous cannulae.
- Urgent blood samples: full blood count, Kleihauer (if woman is rhesus-negative), coagulation studies including fibrinogen, cross-match 4 units of blood (consider asking haematologist to send group-specific blood until cross-matched blood is available).
- Rapid fluid resuscitation with 2 litres of crystalloid.
- Assess need for blood products.
- Use O-negative blood (from labour ward fridge) if there is a life-threatening haemorrhage and consider early use of coagulation products, especially if operative delivery is indicated.
- Assess fetal wellbeing – auscultate the fetal heart or perform an ultrasound scan and commence continuous electronic fetal monitoring if appropriate.

> **An ultrasound scan will fail to detect up to 75% of cases of abruption and therefore time should not be wasted attempting to identify a retroplacental clot using ultrasound scanning.**

ASSESSMENT – rapid evaluation of maternal and fetal condition

Quickly assess the overall condition of the mother and fetus. This includes:

- Ascertain relevant obstetric and clinical history, including:
  - ☐ gestational age
  - ☐ previous uterine surgery/caesarean section
  - ☐ position of placenta (refer to any antenatal scans)
  - ☐ abdominal pain.
- Examination:
  - ☐ estimation of blood loss (see Figure 8.1, page 120)
  - ☐ uterine palpation for tone and tenderness
  - ☐ abdominal palpation for peritonism and ex utero fetal parts
  - ☐ assess placental site using ultrasound scan
  - ☐ once placenta praevia has been excluded, perform a speculum examination to assess degree of bleeding and possible local causes (trauma, polyps, ectropion); consider a vaginal examination to ascertain stage of labour.

> **Remember: do not perform a vaginal examination in the presence of vaginal bleeding without first excluding placenta praevia.**

STOP THE BLEEDING – should birth be expedited?

In cases of massive APH, birth of the baby and placenta is the most effective method of controlling the bleeding, irrespective of the cause, and can be a life-saving intervention for the mother.[8]

If there is a placenta praevia, removal of the abnormally situated placenta should control the bleeding, but the team must be alert to the possibility that there is also a high risk of major PPH. The procedure should be performed by the most experienced obstetrician available and the consultant obstetrician should be in attendance.

If an APH is caused by uterine rupture, the dehiscence should be identified and repaired.

Regardless of the suspected fetal compromise, the maternal condition should always take precedence. If birth is indicated (irrespective of the gestation), the mother should be appropriately resuscitated, and the birth expedited. It should not be delayed for fetal reasons, such as waiting for steroid effect in cases of prematurity.

The neonatal team should be called early in cases of major APH, to ensure adequate time to prepare neonatal resuscitation equipment. APH can cause neonatal anaemia, particularly when there is vasa praevia or abruption.

In cases of major APH it is likely that the birth will be expedited by emergency caesarean section unless the woman is in labour and fully dilated. A caesarean section for major APH (whether caused by a placental abruption, praevia or uterine rupture) is likely to be technically difficult and should be performed by the most experienced obstetrician available. If not already present, the consultant obstetrician should be asked to attend as soon as possible.[8]

The choice of anaesthetic for an operative procedure will depend on the clinical circumstances and maternal condition and should be decided by an experienced anaesthetist.

Finally, an APH is a major risk factor for PPH and, therefore, all members of the team should be prepared to manage any subsequent PPH.

Postpartum haemorrhage

In the UK, major PPH (> 1000 ml) complicates 1.3% of deliveries.[9] The clinical features of shock are as previously described in Table 8.1 (page 119). Major PPH is an obstetric emergency.

Risk factors for major PPH

Prelabour and intrapartum risk factors for PPH are listed in Box 8.1.

Prevention of PPH

There is a strong evidence base to support routine active management of the third stage of labour.[10]

The use of intramuscular Syntometrine® (Alliance) – oxytocin and ergometrine – reduces the risk of PPH by 60%. However, Syntometrine is associated with postpartum hypertension, nausea and vomiting. Oxytocin alone (Syntocinon®; Alliance) is now considered by some authorities to be the agent of choice for women without risk factors for PPH.[4]

Syntocinon given intramuscularly at a dose of 10 units (or 5 units intravenously) is slightly less effective at reducing initial blood loss. However, it is not associated with postpartum hypertension and therefore should be used instead of Syntometrine in the presence of maternal hypertension or if the maternal blood pressure is not known prior to delivery.[11]

> **Syntometrine should not be administered in the presence of known hypertension or if the maternal blood pressure has not been taken during labour.**

Box 8.1 Risk factors for PPH

Prelabour

Previous retained placenta or PPH (recurrence rate of about 8–10%)

Previous caesarean section (associated with placenta praevia, percreta and accreta)

Placenta praevia, accreta or percreta

Antepartum haemorrhage – especially from placental abruption

Overdistension of uterus (e.g. multiple pregnancy, polyhydramnios, macrosomia)

Pre-eclampsia

Body mass index > 35

Increased maternal age (in addition, older women are less tolerant of the effects of a massive bleed)

Existing uterine abnormalities (e.g. fibroids)

Maternal haemoglobin below 9 g/dl at start of labour (less able to tolerate haemorrhage)

Grand multiparity

Intrapartum

Induction of labour

Prolonged first, second or third stage of labour

Oxytocin use in labour

Retained placenta

Precipitate labour

Operative vaginal birth

Caesarean section, particularly in the second stage of labour

Placental abruption

Pyrexia in labour

Uterine atony should be anticipated in clinical situations such as prolonged labour or second-stage caesarean section. In high-risk cases, consideration should be given to administering a longer-acting oxytocic (such as carbetocin 100 micrograms intravenously after caesarean section), or commencing an infusion of Syntocinon 40 units in 500 ml 0.9% saline given intravenously (125 ml/hour) for up to 4 hours after birth in addition to Syntometrine (if appropriate) or Syntocinon.

The 2005–08 Confidential Enquiry into Maternal and Child Deaths[3] and the RCOG[4] recommend that women who have had a previous caesarean section should have their placental site determined by ultrasound; if the placenta is low, magnetic resonance imaging (MRI) can be used together with ultrasound scanning to attempt to determine whether the placenta is accreta or percreta. If either is confirmed, forward planning in the antenatal period and the involvement of an experienced multidisciplinary team at delivery may prevent or reduce the risk of intrapartum and postpartum haemorrhage.[3,4]

Causes of PPH

Major PPH usually occurs within the first hour after delivery. The most common cause is an atonic uterus (70–90%), with or without retained placental tissue.

Genital tract trauma is the next most common cause of PPH, followed by coagulation defects, which are rare but may occur as a result of significant haemorrhage. Table 8.3 lists some of the presenting features, which may be accompanied by signs and symptoms of shock. It is important to remember that bleeding may also be concealed. Concealed heamorrhage should be suspected when the observations and estimated blood loss do not tally.

Rupture of the uterus usually occurs before or at the time of birth, but the diagnosis may not be made until after birth.

Morbid adherence of the placenta to the myometrium (placenta percreta or accreta) is usually diagnosed when massive haemorrhage occurs following unsuccessful attempts to separate and remove the placenta. A case–control study of peripartum hysterectomy carried out by the United Kingdom Obstetric Surveillance System (UKOSS) reported that, of the women requiring peripartum hysterectomy because of haemorrhage, 39% had a morbidly adherent placenta.[12]

Table 8.3 Presenting features and causes of PPH

Presenting feature	Condition of uterus	Possible cause
Vaginal bleeding, placenta complete	'Boggy' and high	Uterine atony
Vaginal bleeding, placenta incomplete	'Boggy' and high	Retained placental tissue
Vaginal bleeding, placenta complete	Well contracted	Vaginal/cervical/perineal trauma
Symptoms of shock, often without vaginal bleeding	Seen at vulva/not palpable abdominally	Inverted uterus
Continual bleeding, blood not clotting, oozing from wound sites	'Boggy' or contracted	Coagulopathy

Initial management of major PPH

The management of a major PPH also requires the prompt initiation of multiple simultaneous actions in a similar sequence to APH. The exact sequence will be dictated by the needs of the individual mother and the resources available.

An outline of the initial management for a major PPH is shown in Figure 8.4. This is discussed in more detail in the following section.

CALL FOR HELP

Activate the emergency buzzer to summon assistance and emergency call the appropriate personnel:

- senior midwife
- experienced obstetrician
- additional support staff
- consultant obstetrician
- consultant anaesthetist
- porter ready to take urgent samples.

Alert the haematologist, blood bank technician and theatre staff to be on standby as the code red major obstetric haemorrhage protocol may be activated.

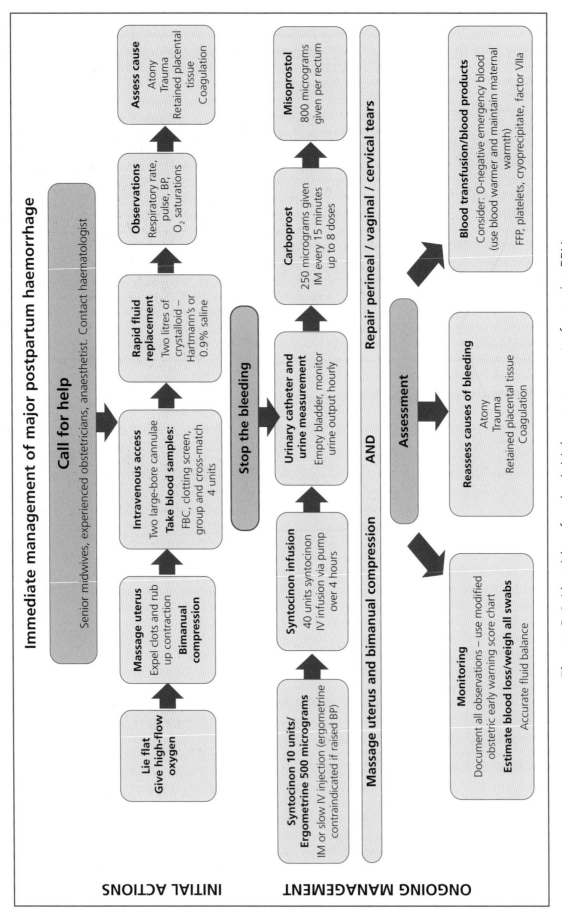

Figure 8.4 Algorithm for the initial management of a major PPH

PPH emergency box

Many units have a PPH emergency box (Figure 8.5) containing emergency equipment, treatment algorithms and medication required for the immediate management of PPH.

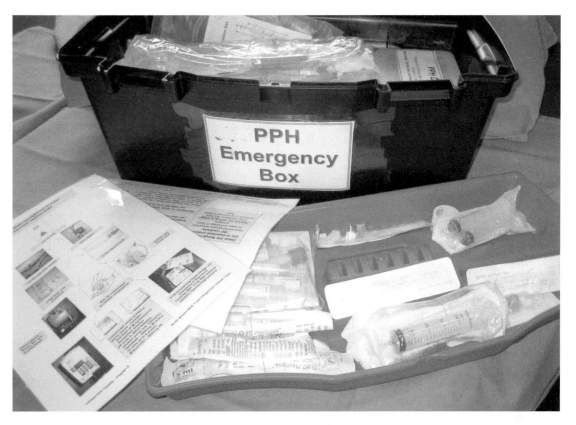

Figure 8.5 The postpartum haemorrhage emergency box

IMMEDIATE ACTIONS – irrespective of cause

- Lie the woman flat and give high-flow facial oxygen.
- Rub up a contraction, expel any clots from the uterus
- Site two large intravenous cannulae and send urgent blood samples: full blood count, coagulation studies including fibrinogen, cross-match 4 units of blood (consider asking haematologist to send group-specific blood until cross-matched blood available).
- Rapid fluid resuscitation of at least 2 litres of crystalloid (e.g. Hartmann's solution or normal saline).
- Autotransfuse by elevation of the mother's legs and/or head-down tilt.
- Use O-negative blood (from labour ward fridge) in cases of life-threatening haemorrhage.

ASSESSMENT – rapid evaluation

Quickly assess the overall condition of the mother. This includes:

- pulse, blood pressure, respiratory rate and oxygen saturations
- peripheral perfusion
- check uterine tone
- estimation of blood loss: weigh swabs, incontinence pads, etc.

Observe for signs of shock:

- maternal tachycardia of greater than 100 beats/minute
- respiratory rate of over 30 breaths/minute
- peripheral vasoconstriction.

All indicate significant blood loss with initial physiological compensation (see Table 8.1; page 119). If the systolic blood pressure falls to less than 100 mmHg, the blood loss is likely to be at least 25% of the maternal blood volume.

Try to identify the cause:

- Check whether the uterus is well contracted.
- Check that the placenta has been expelled and is complete.
- Examine the cervix, vagina and perineum for tears.
- Observe for signs of clotting disorders, such as oozing from wound and cannula sites.

STOP THE BLEEDING

Remember that there may be more than one cause for the bleeding.

Massage the uterus

The most common cause of PPH is uterine atony. Check that the uterus is well contracted – it should feel like 'a cricket ball'. If the uterus is flaccid, 'rub up' a contraction. Expel any blood clots trapped in the uterus, as these inhibit effective uterine contractions. Use bimanual compression if bleeding continues.

First-line drug therapy

If the third stage has not been actively managed, give an oxytocic: either 10 mg oxytocin intramuscularly or 1 ampoule of Syntometrine (oxytocin 5 units and ergometrine 0.5 mg), depending on clinical circumstances and availability.

If an oxytocic has already been given for active management of the third stage but bleeding is continuing, give a second dose of oxytocin as outlined above.

> **Bolus doses of intravenous Syntocinon should be used with caution when there is extreme maternal hypotension, as it can cause a further fall in blood pressure.[13]**

If the uterus contracts with the measures outlined above, a Syntocinon infusion (Syntocinon 40 units diluted in 500 ml physiological saline and infused via an infusion pump at 125 ml/hour over 4 hours) should be commenced to maintain firm uterine tone. However, if the uterine tone is poor, other treatments (e.g. expulsion of blood clots or removal of retained placental tissue) will be required to encourage the uterus to contract, before a Syntocinon infusion will be effective.

Catheterise the bladder

A full bladder can inhibit effective contraction of the uterus. Insert an indwelling Foley catheter to empty the bladder. Note the amount drained and monitor further urinary output hourly as an indicator of renal function.

Repair any tears

Tears of the birth canal can be a source of significant blood loss and are the second most frequent cause of PPH. Apply pressure as an initial holding measure. Stabilise the mother and repair any tears as soon as possible, ensuring adequate analgesia and good lighting. Consider early transfer to theatre, as a full examination under anaesthesia is often required.

Have early recourse to seeking extra help.

Continuing bleeding

Most cases of haemorrhage will be successfully controlled by the simple measures outlined above: a second dose of oxytocin, bladder catheterisation and repair of vaginal tears. However, in some cases the bleeding will not stop and further management is required. This management is most effectively performed in the operating theatre.

Bimanual compression of uterus

If bleeding continues, bimanual compression of the uterus should be performed (Figure 8.6) while the woman is transferred into hospital via ambulance, or transferred to the operating theatre. Bimanual compression is an excellent holding measure and should be continued until the haemorrhage is brought under control.

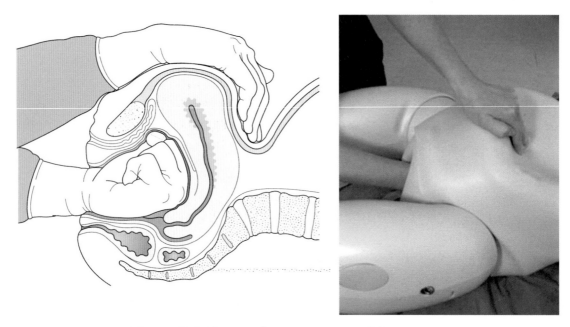

Figure 8.6 Bimanual compression of the uterus

To perform bimanual compression, gently insert one hand into the vagina and form a fist. Direct your fist into the anterior fornix and apply pressure against the anterior wall of the uterus. With the other hand, press externally on the uterine fundus and compress the uterus between your hands. Maintain compression until bleeding is controlled and the uterus contracts.

In the community setting or when a woman is on a postnatal ward, bimanual compression provides an effective mechanical holding measure until arrival on the labour ward.

Examination under anaesthetic

There should be a low threshold for examination under anaesthetic.

Manual removal of retained products

Persistent uterine atony is often caused by retained placental tissue or blood clots. Exploration and emptying of the uterus should be performed as soon as the mother has been resuscitated. This is best performed in the operating theatre and should be done as soon as possible. When the uterus has been manually explored and emptied, further oxytocics should be administered to contract the uterus.

Repair of cervical, vaginal and perineal tears

Adequate analgesia, good lighting and an assistant in theatre make the identification and repair of genital tract tears easier. A systematic approach should be used to ensure that no tears (especially high vaginal and cervical tears) are missed during suturing.

Treatment of unrelenting haemorrhage

Almost all cases of haemorrhage will be controlled by emptying the uterus, giving simple uterotonics and suturing any tears. However, if bleeding continues despite these actions, further management will be required as unrelenting haemorrhage poses a significant threat to the life of the mother.

In cases of unrelenting haemorrhage, both bimanual compression and aortic compression can be used to stem the bleeding until other methods have had time to take effect.

To achieve aortic compression, the aorta must be compressed against the spine. Use a closed fist to apply downward pressure over the abdominal aorta just above and slightly to the left of the umbilicus (Figure 8.7). The femoral pulse should be obliterated if the compression is adequate. This method is especially useful if the PPH occurs during a caesarean section.

The methods used to stop the bleeding will depend largely on the underlying cause of the haemorrhage, but various techniques that should be considered are outlined below.

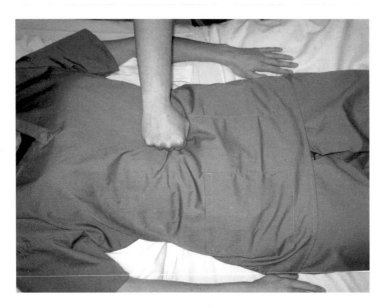

Figure 8.7 Aortic compression

Drug treatments

Carboprost

If the uterus continues to relax despite initial measures, give carboprost (Hemabate®, Pharmacia) 250 micrograms by deep intramuscular injection. This can be repeated at intervals of at least 15 minutes up to a maximum of eight doses.

Adverse effects are uncommon but carboprost can induce vomiting, diarrhoea, headache, hypertension and bronchospasm. Carboprost is contraindicated in mothers with cardiac or pulmonary disease, including asthma.

> **Do not give carboprost intravenously.**
> **Prostaglandins can be fatal if given intravenously.**

Misoprostol

The use of rectal misoprostol (800–1000 micrograms) has been described. Misoprostol is a synthetic analogue of prostaglandin E1 and has the advantage of being thermostable and inexpensive.

A systematic review of the prophylactic use of oral misoprostol for the management of the third stage of labour found that misoprostol 600 micrograms was less effective than conventional uterotonics.[14,15] In situations where conventional uterotonics are available, these should be used in preference to misoprostol. However, misoprostol may be used if first- and second-line uterotonics (e.g. oxytocin, ergometrine and carboprost) are not available or are contraindicated.[4]

Tranexamic acid

Tranexamic acid is an antifibrinolytic that is used widely to prevent and treat haemorrhage in non-obstetric patients. A systematic review published in 2010 suggests that 0.5 g or 1 g tranexamic acid intravenously decreases postpartum blood loss after vaginal birth and after caesarean section.[16] However, further investigations are needed to confirm the efficacy and safety of this regimen. The World Maternal Antifibrinolytic (WOMAN) trial is currently under way and is aiming to provide reliable evidence as to whether tranexamic acid reduces mortality, hysterectomy and other morbidities in women with clinically diagnosed PPH.[17]

Recombinant factor VIIa

Recombinant factor VIIa (rFVIIa) was originally developed for patients with haemophilia. rFVIIa induces haemostasis by enhancing thrombin generation and providing the formation of a stable fibrin clot that is resistant to premature fibrinolysis. Subsequently, it has been used for massive intraoperative haemorrhages.

rFVIIa has been successfully used in obstetrics to control haemorrhage.[18] However, rFVIIa is associated with a high rate of thromboembolic events in patients who receive it. Therefore, it should be used with caution and only after consultation with a consultant haematologist.

The recommended dose is between 40 and 90 micrograms/kg.[4,18] rFVIIa is not effective if platelets and fibrinogen are very low, as these are essential for clot formation. Therefore, before rFVIIa is given, platelets and fibrinogen must be checked and be above 20 x 10^9/l and 1 g/l, respectively.

Mechanical and surgical measures

Laparotomy

If the abdomen is not already open and the bleeding is continuing, a laparotomy may be needed so that surgical methods can be used in an attempt to stop the bleeding. The NICE intrapartum care guideline states that no particular surgical procedure can be recommended above another for the treatment of PPH.[19]

B-Lynch suture and other compression measures

The B-Lynch suture technique is simple and effective with successful outcomes in a number of case reports.[4,20] However, it is not a panacea; in the UKOSS survey, 16% of peripartum hysterectomies performed in the UK were preceded by an unsuccessful B-Lynch or other brace suture.[12]

A simple diagram of the B-Lynch technique is shown in Figure 8.8. The original description of the technique requires the uterine cavity to be opened and explored and a bimanual compression test employed prior to insertion of the suture. If bimanual compression is ineffective in reducing the bleeding, the B-Lynch suture is unlikely to be successful.

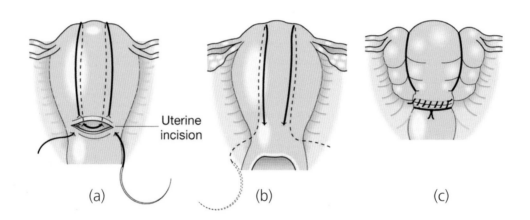

Figure 8.8 The B-Lynch suture: (a) and (b) show the anterior and posterior views of the uterus showing the application of the brace suture; (c) shows the anatomical appearance after complete application (original illustration by Mr Philip Wilson FMAA AIMI, based on the author's video record of the operation; reproduced with permission from *Br J Obstet Gynaecol* 1997;104:374)

More recently, many modifications of the B-Lynch suture have been described. They all follow the same principle of compressing the uterus to stop the bleeding. Some techniques do not require opening of the uterine cavity, while others describe parallel or vertical sutures that compress the anterior uterine wall against the posterior wall.[4] Most of the published series have favourable outcomes, with subsequent pregnancies reported after the procedure. However, serious complications including uterine necrosis[21] and uterine rupture in a subsequent pregnancy[22] have also been reported.

Uterine packing/tamponade

Uterine packing involves completely and uniformly packing the uterine cavity with mesh gauze. The pack can be inserted inside a sterile plastic drape for easier removal. The evidence from many case reports over several decades suggests that uterine packing can be useful in the control of haemorrhage, with few reports of infection or adverse events.[23]

Uterine balloon tamponade (e.g. Bakri [© Cook Medical] or Rusch balloon) can be used in preference to gauze packing. The balloon catheter is inserted into the uterine cavity and inflated with approximately 500 ml of warm saline. An oxytocin infusion may be used to maintain uterine contraction. This method has been described as the 'tamponade test'.[24] If the tamponade test fails to stop the bleeding (following vaginal delivery), a laparotomy will be indicated.

The balloon can be left in place for up to 24 hours. The balloon should ideally be removed in daylight hours when senior staff are available in case bleeding recurs.[4]

Interventional radiology

Interventional radiology should be considered in high-risk cases (e.g. cases of placenta praevia with accreta) where intra-arterial balloons can be placed immediately prior to a planned caesarean section.[4] However, the technique is often difficult to perform in an emergency situation owing to the specialised equipment and personnel required. Therefore, other techniques (e.g. uterine balloon tamponade or compression sutures) may be more appropriate.

Interventional radiology may be particularly useful if there is prolonged or continuous bleeding, once initial treatment has been given and when the mother is stable enough for transfer.

Uterine vessel and internal iliac artery ligation

The uterine ovarian and internal iliac vessels can all be ligated in an attempt to stem uterine bleeding. These are potentially difficult procedures and the assistance of a vascular surgeon should be requested by those inexperienced in the technique.

It is impossible to assess which of the various 'surgical' haemostatic techniques is most effective. Nevertheless, the available observational data suggest that balloon tamponade and haemostatic suturing (e.g. B-Lynch) may be more effective than internal iliac artery ligation and are also easier to perform.[4]

Hysterectomy

Hysterectomy may be necessary if bleeding persists. The incidence of peripartum hysterectomy in the UK in 2005–2006 was 41/100 000 births.[12] It is good practice to involve a second senior doctor (such as a consultant) in the decision for hysterectomy;[4] however, this should not result in unnecessary delay. Furthermore, this course of action should not be delayed by attempts with other unfamiliar techniques.

Unrelenting haemorrhage is probably one of the most testing situations for all professionals involved. While the decision to perform a hysterectomy is never taken lightly, it is important not to delay this course of action until the mother is moribund or the clotting has deteriorated.

Continuing management key points

- Carboprost by deep intramuscular injection.
- Use manual holding measures while arranging further treatment.
- Invasive monitoring.
- Early recourse to surgical intervention.
- Watch out for consumptive coagulopathy.
- Hysterectomy is life saving and should not be delayed
- Aftercare in high-dependency or intensive care unit.

Documentation and high-dependency care

It is important that the woman's clinical response to measures to control haemorrhage and fluid replacement are regularly observed, documented and evaluated. The continuous monitoring of respirations, pulse rate, blood pressure and oxygenation should be commenced. The volume and type of fluid administered should be documented so that fluid balance can be easily monitored. The maternal temperature should be regularly monitored as hypothermia can easily develop from the administration of non-warmed blood products.

Clinical observations and fluid balance should be plotted on a high-dependency chart which includes modified obstetric early warning scores for early recognition of any deterioration in condition.[3]

High-dependency care

Women who have experienced major obstetric haemorrhage (antepartum or postpartum) that causes maternal compromise require high-dependency care.

Central venous pressure monitoring at an early stage, to guide fluid replacement, has been emphasised in the Confidential Enquiries into Maternal Deaths.[3] This may be particularly useful when major haemorrhage occurs in a woman with pre-eclampsia, where there is a fine balance between fluid replacement and fluid overload.

Some women may need to be transferred to the intensive therapy unit (ITU), either because of a need for specialist monitoring/therapy or if labour ward staff are unable to deliver supportive care. It is important for the multi-professional team to involve intensivists at an early stage to prevent delay in admission to the ITU. The use of a maternal SBAR form may aid the communication process for transfer between labour ward and ITU (see **Module 1**, Figure 1.1, page 5 for an example of maternal SBAR form).

References

1. Khan KS, Wojdyla D, Say L, Gülmezoglu AM, Van Look PF. WHO analysis of causes of maternal death: a systematic review. *Lancet* 2006;367:1066–74.

2. Brace V, Kernaghan D, Penney G. Learning from adverse clinical outcomes: major obstetric haemorrhage in Scotland, 2003–05. *BJOG* 2007;114:1388–96.

3. Centre for Maternal and Child Enquiries. Saving Mothers' Lives: reviewing maternal deaths to make motherhood safer: 2006–08. The Eighth Report in Confidential Enquiries into Maternal Deaths in the United Kingdom. *BJOG* 2011;118 Suppl 1:1–203.

4. Royal College of Obstetricians and Gynaecologists. *Prevention and Management of Postpartum Haemorrhage*. Green-top Guideline No. 52. London: RCOG; 2009 [www.rcog.org.uk/womens-health/clinical-guidance/prevention-and-management-postpartum-haemorrhage-green-top-52].

5. Schierhout G, Roberts I. Fluid resuscitation with colloid or crystalloid solutions in critically ill patients: a systematic review of randomised trials. *BMJ* 1998;316:961–4.

6. Mittermayr M, Streif W, Haas T, Fries D, Velik-Salchner C, Klingler A, et al. Hemostatic changes after crystalloid or colloid fluid administration during major orthopedic surgery: the role of fibrinogen administration. *Anesth Analg* 2007;105:905–17.

7. James DK, Steer PJ, Weiner CP, Gonik B, Crowther C, Robson S. *High Risk Pregnancy: Management Options*. 4th edition. St Louis: Elsevier; 2010.

8. Royal College Obstetricians and Gynaecologists. *Antepartum Haemorrhage*. Green-top

Guideline No. 63. London; 2011 [www.rcog.org.uk/womens-health/clinical-guidance/antepartum-haemorrhage-green-top-63].

9. Stones RW, Paterson CM, Saunders NJ. Risk factors for major obstetric haemorrhage. *Eur J Obstet Gynecol Reprod Biol* 1993;48:15–8.

10. McDonald S, Prendiville WJ, Elbourne D. Prophylactic ergometriene–oxytocin versus oxytocin for the third stage of labour. *Cochrane Database Syst Rev* 2004;(1):CD000201.

11. Lewis G (editor). The Confidential Enquiry into Maternal and Child Health (CEMACH). *Saving Mothers' Lives: Reviewing Maternal Deaths to Make Motherhood Safer 2003–2005. The Seventh Report on Confidential Enquiries into Maternal Deaths in the United Kingdom.* London: CEMACH; 2007.

12. Knight M, Kurinczuk JJ, Spark P, Brocklehurst P; United Kingdom Surveillance System Steering Committee. Cesarean delivery and peripartum hysterectomy. *Obstet Gynecol* 2008;111:97–105.

13. Lewis G (editor). The Confidential Enquiry into Maternal and Child Health (CEMACH). *Why Mothers Die 2000–2003. The Sixth Report on Confidential Enquiries into Maternal Deaths in the United Kingdom.* London: RCOG Press; 2004.

14. Gülmezoglu AM, Forna F, Villar J, Hofmeyr GJ. Prostaglandins for prevention of postpartum haemorrhage. *Cochrane Database Syst Rev* 2004;(1):CD000494.

15. Mousa HA, Alfirevic Z. Treatment for primary postpartum haemorrhage. *Cochrane Database Syst Rev* 2007;(1):CD003249.

16. Novikova N, Hofmeyr GJ. Tranexamic acid for preventing postpartum haemorrhage. *Cochrane Database Syst Rev* 2010;(7):CD007872.

17. Shakur H, Elbourne D, Gülmezoglu M, Alfirevic Z, Ronsmans C, Allen E, et al. The WOMAN Trial (World Maternal Antifibrinolytic Trial): tranexamic acid for the treatment of postpartum haemorrhage: an international randomised, double blind placebo controlled trial. *Trials* 2010;11:40.

18. Franchini M, Lippi G, Franchi M. The use of recombinant activated factor VII in obstetric and gynaecological haemorrhage. *BJOG* 2007;114:8–15.

19. National Collaborating Centre for Women's and Children's Health. *Intrapartum care: care of healthy women and their babies durng childbirth.* London: RCOG; 2007.

20. B-Lynch C, Coker A, Lawal AH, Abu J, Cowen MJ. The B-Lynch surgical technique for the control of massive postpartum haemorrhage: an alternative to hysterectomy? Five cases reported. *Br J Obstet Gynaecol* 1997;104:372–5.

21. Treloar EJ, Anderson RS, Andrews HS, Bailey JL. Uterine necrosis following B-Lynch suture for primary postpartum haemorrhage. *BJOG* 2006;113:486–8.

22. Pechtor K, Richards B, Paterson H. Antenatal catastrophic uterine rupture at 32 weeks of gestation after previous B-Lynch suture. *BJOG* 2010;117:889–91.

23. Maier RC. Control of postpartum hemorrhage with uterine packing. *Am J Obstet Gynecol* 1993;169:317–21; discussion 321–3.

24. Frenzel D, Condous GS, Papageorghiou AT, McWhinney NA. The use of the "tamponade test" to stop massive obstetric haemorrhage in placenta accreta. *BJOG* 2005;112:676–7.

Module 9
Shoulder dystocia

Key learning points

- Shoulder dystocia is unpredictable.
- Understand that only **routine axial traction** should be applied.
- Understand manoeuvres required to effect birth during shoulder dystocia.
- Understand the importance of clear and accurate documentation.
- Awareness of potential complications of shoulder dystocia.

Common difficulties observed in training drills

- Not calling the neonatologist.
- Failing to state the problem.
- Inability to gain appropriate internal vaginal access.
- Confusion over internal rotational manoeuvres.
- Resorting to excessive traction to effect birth.
- Use of fundal pressure.

Introduction

Definition

Shoulder dystocia is when additional manoeuvres (such as McRoberts' position and suprapubic pressure) are required to complete the birth of the baby, after routine traction has failed to release the shoulders during a normal vaginal birth.[1]

Incidence

There is wide variation in the reported incidence of shoulder dystocia.[2] Studies involving the largest number of vaginal births report incidences between 0.58% and 0.70%.[3–8]

Pathophysiology

When shoulder dystocia occurs, the anterior fetal shoulder impacts on the maternal symphysis pubis after birth of the head, preventing birth of the body (Figure 9.1). Less commonly, the posterior fetal shoulder impacts on the maternal sacral promontory.

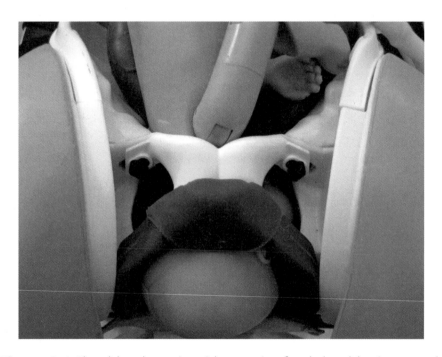

Figure 9.1 Shoulder dystocia with anterior fetal shoulder impacted on maternal symphysis pubis

Risk factors for shoulder dystocia

A number of antenatal and intrapartum characteristics have been reported to be associated with shoulder dystocia (Box 9.1), but even a combination of risk factors is poorly predictive.[9,10] Conventional risk factors predicted only 16% of cases of shoulder dystocia that resulted in infant morbidity.[11]

Box 9.1 Risk factors for shoulder dystocia	
Prelabour	**Intrapartum**
Previous shoulder dystocia	Prolonged first stage
Macrosomia	Prolonged second stage
Maternal diabetes mellitus	Labour augmentation
Maternal obesity	Instrumental delivery

Previous shoulder dystocia is a risk factor for recurrent shoulder dystocia. The rate of shoulder dystocia in women who have had shoulder dystocia in a previous birth has been reported to be 10 times higher than the rate in the general population.[12] However, this may be an underestimate, as caesarean section rates are higher following severe shoulder dystocia.

Macrosomia

Large fetal size increases the risk of shoulder dystocia: the greater the fetal birth weight, the higher the risk of shoulder dystocia. A review of 14 721 births reported rates of shoulder dystocia in non-diabetic mothers of 1% in infants weighing less than 4000 g, 10% in infants weighing 4000–4499 g and 23% in infants weighing more than 4500 g.[13] However, macrosomia remains a weak predictor of shoulder dystocia. The large majority of infants with a birth weight of greater than 4500 g do not develop shoulder dystocia and up to 50% of cases of shoulder dystocia occur in infants with a birth weight less than 4000 g.[4] Furthermore, antenatal detection of macrosomia is poor: third-trimester ultrasound scans have at least a 10% margin of error for actual birth weight and detect only 60% of infants weighing over 4500 g.[14]

Maternal diabetes mellitus

Maternal diabetes mellitus increases the risk of shoulder dystocia.[9] Infants of diabetic mothers have a two- to four-fold increased risk of shoulder dystocia compared with infants of the same birth weight born to non-diabetic mothers.[9,15] This is probably attributable to the different body shape of babies born to diabetic mothers.

Instrumental delivery

There is a higher rate of shoulder dystocia associated with instrumental birth than with a normal vaginal birth.[16]

Obesity

Women with a raised body mass index (BMI) are at higher risk of shoulder dystocia than women with a normal BMI.[17] However, women who are obese tend to have larger babies and the association between maternal obesity and shoulder dystocia is therefore likely to be attributable to fetal macrosomia, rather than the maternal obesity itself.[18]

Key points

- The majority of cases of shoulder dystocia occur in women with no risk factors.
- Shoulder dystocia is therefore an unpredictable and largely unpreventable event.
- Clinicians should be aware of existing risk factors but must always be alert to the possibility of shoulder dystocia with any birth.

Prevention

Shoulder dystocia can only be prevented by caesarean section. However, even in the presence of suspected fetal macrosomia, elective caesarean section is not recommended as a method of reducing potential morbidity from possible shoulder dystocia. It has been estimated that an additional 2345 caesarean births would be required to prevent one permanent injury from shoulder dystocia.[14]

Elective caesarean section is recommended for women with diabetes and suspected fetal macrosomia (> 4.5 kg) or where the estimated fetal weight is greater than 5 kg in a woman without diabetes.[19] This is because of the higher incidence of shoulder dystocia and brachial plexus injury in this subgroup.

Management

There are numerous manoeuvres that can be used to resolve shoulder dystocia. The RCOG algorithm for the management of shoulder dystocia is shown in Figure 9.2. This is described in detail in the next section.

There is no evidence that one intervention is superior to another; therefore, the algorithm begins with simple measures that are often effective and leads progressively to manoeuvres that are more invasive. Variations in the sequence of actions may be appropriate.

Recognition of shoulder dystocia

- There may be difficulty with birth of the face and chin.
- When the head is born, it remains tightly applied to the vulva.
- The chin retracts and depresses the perineum – the 'turtle-neck' sign.
- The anterior shoulder fails to release with maternal pushing and/or when routine axial traction is applied.

Call for help

- Use the emergency buzzer (not the call bell).
- Call for:
  - □ senior midwife
  - □ additional midwifery staff
  - □ the most experienced obstetrician available
  - □ neonatologist.
- Remember to call for the neonatologist – this is often forgotten.
- Consider calling the obstetric consultant and an anaesthetist.

Clearly state the problem. Announce 'shoulder dystocia' as help arrives.

Note the time the head was delivered (start the clock on the resuscitaire or mark the CTG, if monitoring).

Ask the mother to stop pushing. Pushing should be discouraged, as it may increase the impaction and therefore the risk of neurological and orthopaedic complications, and will not resolve the dystocia.

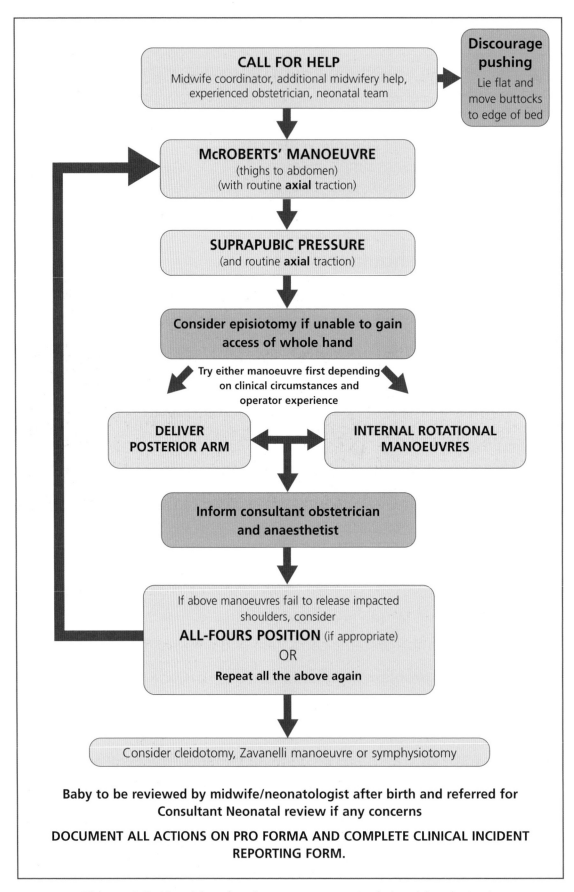

Figure 9.2 Algorithm for the management of shoulder dystocia

McRoberts' manoeuvre

The McRoberts' manoeuvre is an effective intervention with reported success rates as high as 90%.[19] It has a low rate of complication and is one of the least invasive manoeuvres, and therefore, if possible, should be employed first.

Lie the mother flat and remove any pillows from under her back. Bring her to the end of the bed and/or remove the end of the bed to make vaginal access easier. With one assistant on either side, hyperflex the mother's legs against her abdomen so that her knees are up towards her ears (Figure 9.3). If the mother is in the lithotomy position, her legs will need to be removed from the supports to achieve McRoberts' positioning.

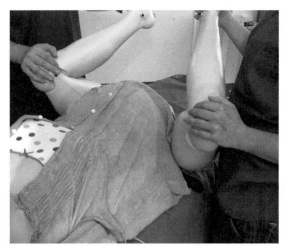 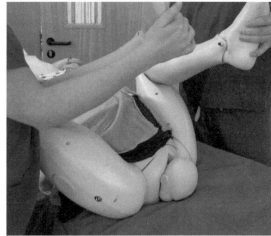

Figure 9.3 McRoberts' position

McRoberts' position increases the relative anteroposterior diameter of the pelvic inlet by rotating the maternal pelvis cephaloid and straightening the sacrum relative to the lumbar spine.

Routine axial traction – the same degree of traction as applied during a normal birth and in an axial direction, i.e. in line with the axis of the fetal spine (Figure 9.4) – should then be applied to the baby's head to assess whether the shoulders have been released.

If the anterior shoulder is not released with McRoberts' position, move on to the next manoeuvre. Do not continue to apply traction to the baby's head.

> **Remember: shoulder dystocia is a 'bony problem' where the baby's shoulder is obstructed by the mother's pelvis. If the entrapment is not released by McRoberts' position, another manoeuvre (not traction) is required to free the shoulder and achieve birth.**

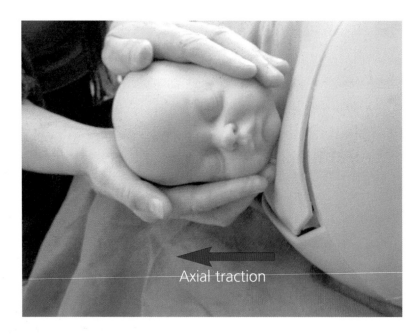

Figure 9.4 Routine axial traction

McRoberts' position performed before birth of the baby's head, in anticipation of shoulder dystocia, is not recommended as a prophylactic manoeuvre as it is ineffective.

Suprapubic pressure

Suprapubic pressure aims to reduce the fetal bisacromial (shoulder-to-shoulder) diameter and rotate the anterior fetal shoulder into the wider oblique diameter of the pelvis. The anterior shoulder is freed to slip underneath the symphysis pubis with the aid of routine axial traction.[20]

An assistant should apply suprapubic pressure from the side of the fetal back (if this is known). Pressure is applied in a downward and lateral direction, just above the maternal symphysis pubis, to push the posterior aspect of the anterior shoulder towards the fetal chest (Figure 9.5). If you are unsure of the location of the fetal back, suprapubic pressure should be applied from the most likely side of the fetal back and, if this is unsuccessful at resolving the dystocia, suprapubic pressure can be attempted from the other side.

There is no evidence that rocking is better than continuous pressure when performing suprapubic pressure, nor that it should be performed for 30 seconds for it to be effective. Only routine axial traction should be applied to the fetal head when assessing whether the manoeuvre has been successful. Again, if the anterior shoulder is not released with suprapubic pressure and routine axial traction, the next manoeuvre should be attempted.

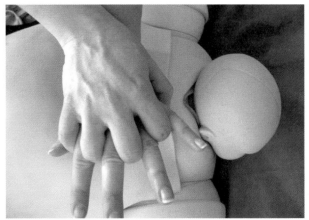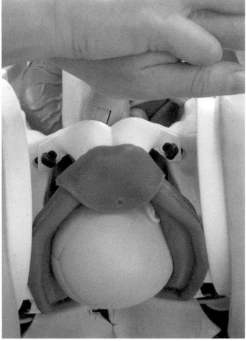

Figure 9.5 Applying suprapubic pressure

Evaluate the need for an episiotomy

An episiotomy will not relieve the bony obstruction of shoulder dystocia but may be required to allow the accoucheur more space to facilitate internal vaginal manoeuvres (delivery of the posterior arm or internal rotation of the shoulders). Often the perineum has already torn or an episiotomy may have already been performed before birth of the head, and with the correct technique there is almost always enough room to gain internal access without performing an episiotomy.[21]

Internal manoeuvres

There are two categories of internal vaginal manoeuvre that can be performed if McRoberts' position and suprapubic pressure have not been effective: internal rotational manoeuvres and delivery of the posterior arm. There is no evidence demonstrating that either manoeuvre is superior or that one should be attempted before the other, but all internal manoeuvres start with the same action: inserting the whole hand posteriorly into the sacral hollow.

Gaining internal vaginal access

When shoulder dystocia occurs, the problem is usually at the inlet of the pelvis, with the anterior shoulder trapped above the symphysis pubis.

The temptation, therefore, is to try to gain vaginal access anteriorly to perform manoeuvres. However, there is very little room underneath the pubic arch and therefore attempting any manoeuvre can be extremely difficult (Figure 9.6).

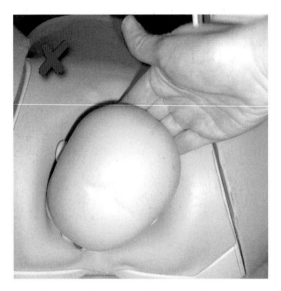

a. Attempting to gain anterior access

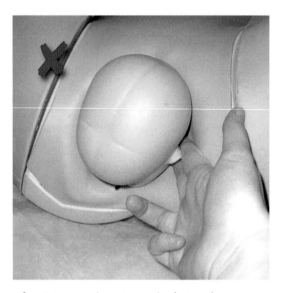

b. Attempting to gain lateral access

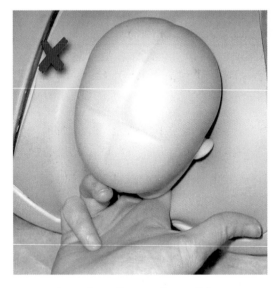

c. Entering the vagina with two fingers as if performing a routine vaginal examination

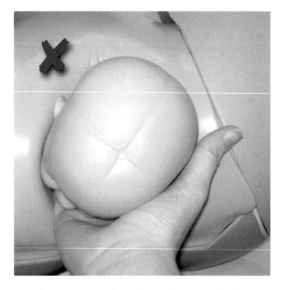

d. Leaving the thumb out of the vagina

Figure 9.6 Incorrect attempts at gaining vaginal access

The most spacious part of the pelvis is in the sacral hollow; therefore, vaginal access can be gained more easily posteriorly, into the sacral hollow. If the accoucheur scrunches up their hand (as if putting on a tight bracelet or reaching for the last Pringles® crisp in the bottom of the container), internal rotation or delivery of the posterior arm can then be attempted using the whole hand (Figure 9.7).

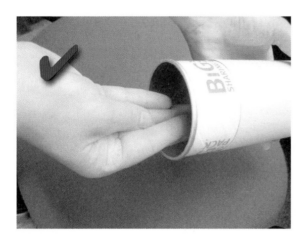 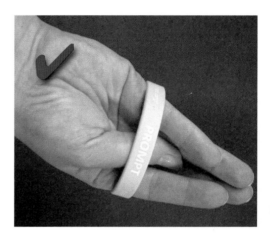

Figure 9.7 Correct vaginal access

Delivery of the posterior arm

Delivering the posterior arm will reduce the diameter of the fetal shoulders by the width of the arm. This will usually provide enough room to resolve the shoulder dystocia.

Often, babies lie with their arms flexed across their chest and so, as your hand enters the vagina posteriorly, you will feel the fetal hand and forearm of the posterior arm (Figure 9.8). In this case, take hold of the fetal wrist (with your fingers and thumb) and gently release the posterior arm in a straight line (Figure 9.9). This movement of the fetal arm is similar to the action of 'putting your hand up in class'. Once the posterior arm is delivered (Figure 9.10), apply gentle axial traction to the fetal head. If the shoulder dystocia has resolved, the baby should then be easily delivered.

If, despite delivering the posterior arm, the shoulder dystocia has not resolved, support the head and posterior arm and gently rotate the baby through 180 degrees. The posterior shoulder will then become the new anterior shoulder and should be below the symphysis pubis, thus resolving the dystocia.

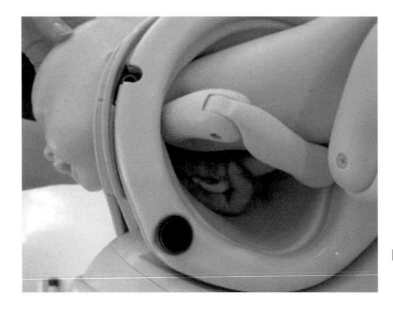

Figure 9.8 Location of the posterior arm

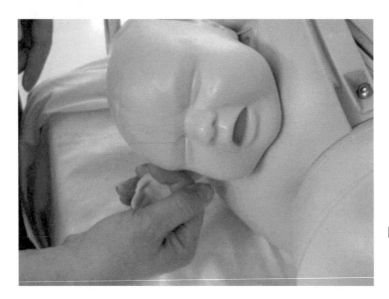

Figure 9.9 Gentle traction on the posterior arm in a straight line

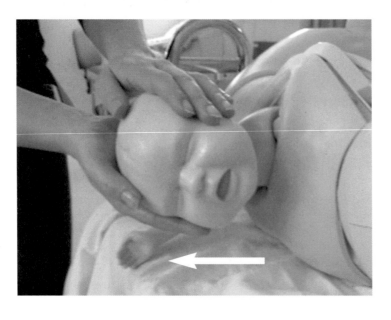

Figure 9.10 Routine axial traction to deliver the rest of the body

If the baby is lying with its posterior arm straight against its body (in front of the fetal abdomen), rather than with a flexed posterior arm, this is much more difficult to deliver. In this situation, it may be easier to attempt internal rotational manoeuvres instead. To deliver a straight posterior arm, the arm needs to be flexed so that the wrist can be grasped. This can be done by the accoucheur following the straight posterior arm down to the elbow, placing their thumb in the antecubital fossa and then applying pressure with their fingers to the back of the forearm just below the elbow. This should flex the posterior arm. The wrist can then be grasped and the arm delivered as previously described. If you cannot reach the wrist, do not pull on the upper arm as this is likely to result in a humeral fracture.

> **Remember to ask for suprapubic pressure to be stopped while you gain internal vaginal access and attempt internal manoeuvres.**

Internal rotational manoeuvres

The aims of internal rotation are:

- to move the fetal shoulders (the bisacromial diameter) out of the narrowest diameter of the mother's pelvis (the anterior–posterior) and into a wider pelvic diameter (the oblique or transverse)
- to use the maternal pelvic anatomy: as the fetal shoulders are rotated within the mother's pelvis, the fetal shoulder descends through the pelvis owing to the bony architecture of the pelvis.

Internal rotational manoeuvres were originally described by Woods and Rubin. Rotation can be most easily achieved by pressing on the anterior (front) or posterior (back) aspect of the posterior (lowermost) shoulder (Figure 9.11). Pressure on the posterior aspect of the posterior shoulder has the added benefit of reducing the shoulder diameter by adducting the shoulders (scrunching the shoulders inwards). Rotation should move the shoulders into the wider oblique diameter, resolving the shoulder dystocia, so that delivery is possible with routine traction. If delivery does not occur, continue the pressure and, by swapping hands, rotate the shoulders a complete turn (180-degree rotation). This manoeuvre (as with rotation after delivery of the posterior arm) substitutes the anterior shoulder for the posterior shoulder and will resolve the dystocia.

If pressure in one direction has no effect, try to rotate the shoulders in the opposite direction by pressing on the other side of the fetal posterior

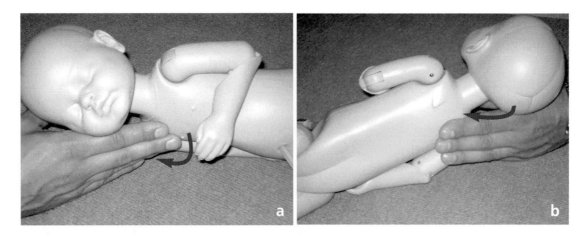

Figure 9.11 Internal rotational manoeuvres: (a) pressure on the anterior aspect of the posterior shoulder to achieve rotation; (b) pressure on the posterior aspect of the posterior shoulder to achieve rotation

shoulder (that is, change from pressing on the front of the baby's shoulder to the back of the baby's shoulder or vice versa). If you are struggling, try changing the hand you are using.

If pressure on the posterior shoulder is unsuccessful, apply pressure on the anterior fetal shoulder. This is more difficult, as it is hard to reach the anterior shoulder. From the sacral hollow, follow the fetal back up to the anterior shoulder. Apply pressure on the posterior aspect of the anterior shoulder to adduct and rotate the shoulders into the oblique diameter.

While attempting to rotate the fetal shoulders from the inside of the pelvis, you can instruct a colleague to perform suprapubic pressure to assist your rotation. Ensure that you are pushing with and not against each other.

All-fours position

The all-fours position has been described to have an 83% success rate in one small case series.[22] Individual circumstances should guide the accoucheur's decision whether to try the all-fours technique before or after attempting internal rotation and delivery of the posterior arm. For a slim mobile woman without epidural anaesthesia and with a single midwifery attendant, the all-fours position is probably more appropriate and clearly this may be a useful option in a community setting. For a less mobile woman with epidural anaesthesia in place, internal manoeuvres are more appropriate.

Roll the mother on to her hands and knees so that the maternal weight lies evenly on the four limbs. This simple change of position may dislodge the anterior shoulder and the woman may spontaneously push, or routine axial traction may be applied to the fetal head, to ascertain if the dystocia has been resolved. If dystocia remains, the all-fours position also facilitates access to the posterior shoulder to enable internal manoeuvres to be performed.

> **Remember when the woman is in an all-fours position that the maternal sacral hollow and the fetal posterior shoulder will both be uppermost.**

Additional manoeuvres

Several last-resort methods have been described for those cases resistant to all standard measures. It is very rare that these are required if the manouevres described previously are performed correctly.

Vaginal replacement of the head (Zavanelli manoeuvre) and then delivery by caesarean section has been described,[23,24] but success rates vary.[25] The maternal safety of this procedure is unknown, however; this should be borne in mind, given that a high proportion of fetuses have irreversible hypoxia–acidosis by this stage. As the uterus will have retracted following delivery of the fetal head, a uterolytic (e.g. terbutaline 0.25 mg subcutaneously or sublingual glyceryl trinitrate) should be given prior to any attempts to replace the fetal head to reduce the risk of uterine rupture.

Symphysiotomy (partial surgical division of the maternal symphysis pubis ligament) has been suggested as a potentially useful procedure. However, there is a high incidence of serious maternal morbidity and poor neonatal outcome.[26] Other techniques, including the use of a posterior axillary sling, have been reported but there are few data available.[27,28]

How much time do I have?

It is not possible to recommend an absolute time limit for the management of shoulder dystocia as the head-to-body birth interval that each individual fetus can withstand without hypoxia occurring will vary depending on clinical circumstances. The condition of the baby at eventual delivery is dependent on the head-to-body interval but also the fetal condition at the start of the dystocia.

A review of fatal cases of shoulder dystocia in the UK reported that 47% of the babies that died did so within 5 minutes of the head being delivered; however, there was a very high proportion of cases in which the fetus had a pathological CTG prior to the shoulder dystocia.[29] A more recent review reported there was a very low rate of hypoxic ischaemic injury if the head-to-body delivery time was less than 5 minutes.[30] However, imposing time limits may cause accoucheurs to resort to more forceful traction as the 5-minute time limit approaches, and therefore it may be better to emphasise the importance of managing the problem as efficiently as possible to avoid hypoxia and as carefully as possible to avoid unnecessary trauma.

What to avoid

Traction

It may be an instinctive reaction to pull on the fetal head in an attempt to assist the birth of the baby. However, traction alone will not resolve the dystocia and **excessive traction should be avoided**.

In addition, traction applied in a downward direction on the fetal head is strongly associated with obstetric brachial plexus injury. Therefore, **downward traction on the fetal head** should be avoided in the management of all births.

There is also some evidence that traction applied quickly with a 'jerk', rather than applied slowly, may be more damaging to the nerves of the brachial plexus[31] (imagine trying to snap a piece of cotton – it is much easier to break it with a quick pull than a slow one).

> **Routine traction should always be applied slowly and gently in an axial direction and not with sudden force or in a downward direction.**

Fundal pressure

Fundal pressure is associated with a high rate of brachial plexus injury and rupture of the uterus. It should therefore **not be applied** during shoulder dystocia.[29]

Documentation

Accurate documentation of a difficult and potentially traumatic delivery is essential. It is important to write a clear explanation of the manoeuvres that were performed, such that someone else reading it could reproduce those actions (it is not essential to use names of manoeuvres). It may be helpful to use a pro forma to aid accurate record keeping. An example is provided in Figure 9.12.

It is important to record:

- the time of delivery of the head
- the manoeuvres performed, the timing and the sequence
- the traction applied
- the time of delivery of the body
- the staff in attendance and the time they arrived
- the condition of the baby
- umbilical cord blood acid–base measurements (cord pH)
- the anterior fetal shoulder at the time of the dystocia.

Parents

Shoulder dystocia is a frightening and potentially traumatic experience for the mother and her attending family. It is important to tell the parents what is happening and to give the mother clear instructions during the emergency. Both the birth and the reason for the use of manoeuvres should be discussed after delivery.

Any baby with a suspected injury following shoulder dystocia should be immediately reviewed by a neonatologist. The Erb's Palsy Group is an excellent source of information and supports families and healthcare practitioners caring for children with brachial plexus injuries (www.erbspalsygroup.co.uk).

A woman who has had a previous shoulder dystocia should be referred to a consultant-led antenatal clinic in subsequent pregnancies to discuss antenatal care and mode of birth.

SHOULDER DYSTOCIA DOCUMENTATION

PROMPT
Making Childbirth Safer, Together

Date .... Time ....

Person completing form ....Designation........

Signature ....

Mother's Name :
Date of birth :
Hospital Number
Consultant

Called for help at:

Staff present at delivery of head:		Additional staff attending for delivery of shoulders		
Name	Role	Name	Role	Time arrived

Procedures used to assist delivery	By whom	Time	Order	Details	Reason if not performed
McRoberts' position:					
Suprapubic pressure:				From maternal **left** / **right** (circle as appropriate)	
Episiotomy:				Not required as enough room for access / perineal tear present /already performed for delivery of head (circle as appropriate)	
Delivery of posterior arm:				**Right** / **left** arm (circle as appropriate)	
Internal rotational manoeuvre:					
Description of rotation:					
Description of traction:	Routine axial (as in normal vaginal birth)	Other -		Reason if not routine	
Other manoeuvres used:					

Mode of delivery of head:	Spontaneous		Instrumental – vacuum / forceps	
Time of delivery of head:	Time of delivery of baby		Head-to-body delivery interval	
Fetal position during dystocia:	Head facing maternal **left** **Left** fetal shoulder anterior		Head facing maternal **right** **Right** fetal shoulder anterior	
Birth weight kg	Apgar	1 min :	5 mins :	10 mins :
Cord gases:	Art pH :	Art BE:	Venous pH :	Venous BE :
Explanation to parents	Yes	By	AIMS form completed	Yes

Neonatologist called: Yes / No   Time arrived: ....   Neonatologists name: ....

Baby assessment at delivery (maybe done by M/W): Any sign of arm weakness? Any sign of potential bony fracture? Baby admitted to Neonatal Intensive Care Unit? Assessment by	Yes Yes Yes	No No No	If yes to any of these questions for review and follow up by Consultant neonatologist

Reproduced with kind permission of North Bristol NHS Trust.

Figure 9.12 An example of a shoulder dystocia documentation pro forma

Consequences of shoulder dystocia

Shoulder dystocia has a high perinatal morbidity and mortality rate.[5] Maternal morbidity is also increased (Box 9.2).

Box 9.2 Perinatal morbidity and mortality	
Perinatal	**Maternal**
Stillbirth	Postpartum haemorrhage
Hypoxia	Third- and fourth-degree tears
Brachial plexus injury	Uterine rupture
Fractures (humeral and clavicular)	Psychological distress

Acidosis

Shoulder dystocia is an acute life-threatening event. A healthy fetus will compensate during shoulder dystocia but only for a finite amount of time. Babies may be born with a severe metabolic acidosis or may develop hypoxic ischaemic encephalopathy (HIE), with or without long-term neurological damage. The necessary resuscitation equipment should therefore be prepared and neonatal staff should be called as soon as shoulder dystocia occurs in case neonatal resuscitation is required.

Brachial plexus injury

Brachial plexus injury is one of the most important complications of shoulder dystocia and it affects approximately 1/2300 deliveries in the UK.[32] The primary mechanism for brachial plexus injury is thought to be excessive traction on the fetal head during shoulder dystocia, although other mechanisms of injury have been proposed. Brachial plexus injury may be a complication of normal labour and has even been reported after caesarean section.

Injuries can be divided into upper (Erb's palsy), lower (Klumpke's palsy) or total brachial plexus injury:

- **Erb's palsy** is the most common injury. The upper arm is flaccid and the lower arm is extended and rotated towards the body with the hand held in a classic 'waiter's tip' posture. Up to 90% of Erb's palsies recover by 12 months.

- **Klumpke's palsy** is less common. The hand is limp, with no movement of the fingers. The recovery rate is lower and around 40% of injuries resolve by 12 months.

- **Total brachial plexus** injury occurs in approximately 20% of brachial plexus injuries. There is a total sensory and motor deficit of the entire arm, making it completely paralysed with no sensation. Horner syndrome, caused by sympathetic nerve injury resulting in contraction of the pupil and ptosis of the eyelid on the affected side, may also be present. Full functional recovery is rare without surgical intervention. The prognosis is worse if Horner syndrome is present.

Humeral and clavicular fractures

Humeral and clavicular fractures can also occur following shoulder dystocia. These fractures usually heal quickly and have a good prognosis.

Shoulder dystocia is an unpredictable obstetric emergency	
Problem	Clearly state the problem
Paediatrician	Immediately call the paediatrician/neonatologist
Position	McRoberts' or all fours
Pressure	Suprapubic (NOT FUNDAL) pressure
Posterior	Vaginal access gained posteriorly
Pringle®	Get the whole hand in
Pull	Don't keep pulling if a manouevre has not worked
Pro forma	Documentation should be clear and concise
Parents	Communication and explanation are essential

References

1. Resnick R. Management of shoulder girdle dystocia. *Clin Obstet Gynecol* 1980;23:559–64.
2. Gherman RB. Shoulder dystocia: an evidence-based evaluation of the obstetric nightmare. *Clin Obstet Gynecol* 2002;45:345–62.
3. McFarland M, Hod M, Piper JM, Xenakis EM, Langer O. Are labor abnormalities more common in shoulder dystocia? *Am J Obstet Gynecol* 1995;173:1211–4.

4. Baskett TF, Allen AC. Perinatal implications of shoulder dystocia. *Obstet Gynecol* 1995;86:14–7.

5. Gherman RB, Ouzounian JG, Goodwin TM. Obstetric maneuvers for shoulder dystocia and associated fetal morbidity. *Am J Obstet Gynecol* 1998;178:1126–30.

6. McFarland MB, Langer O, Piper JM, Berkus MD. Perinatal outcome and the type and number of maneuvers in shoulder dystocia. *Int J Gynaecol Obstet* 1996;55:219–24.

7. Ouzounian JG, Gherman RB. Shoulder dystocia: are historic risk factors reliable predictors? *Am J Obstet Gynecol* 2005;192:1933–5.

8. Smith RB, Lane C, Pearson JF. Shoulder dystocia: what happens at the next delivery? *Br J Obstet Gynaecol* 1994;101:713–5.

9. Nesbitt TS, Gilbert WM, Herrchen B. Shoulder dystocia and associated risk factors with macrosomic infants born in California. *Am J Obstet Gynecol* 1998;179:476–80.

10. Bahar AM. Risk factors and fetal outcome in cases of shoulder dystocia compared with normal deliveries of a similar birthweight. *Br J Obstet Gynaecol* 1996;103:868–72.

11. Gross TL, Sokol RJ, Williams T, Thompson K. Shoulder dystocia: a fetal–physician risk. *Am J Obstet Gynecol* 1987;156:1408–18.

12. Mehta SH, Blackwell SC, Chadha R, Sokol RJ. Shoulder dystocia and the next delivery: outcomes and management. *J Matern Fetal Neonatal Med* 2007;20:729–33.

13. Acker DB, Sachs BP, Friedman EA. Risk factors for shoulder dystocia in the average-weight infant. *Obstet Gynecol* 1986;67:614–8.

14. Rouse DJ, Owen J. Prophylactic cesarean delivery for fetal macrosomia diagnosed by means of ultrasonography – A Faustian bargain? *Am J Obstet Gynecol* 1999;181:332–8.

15. Acker DB, Sachs BP, Friedman EA. Risk factors for shoulder dystocia. *Obstet Gynecol* 1985;66:762–8.

16. Benedetti TJ, Gabbe SG. Shoulder dystocia. A complication of fetal macrosomia and prolonged second stage of labor with midpelvic delivery. *Obstet Gynecol* 1978;52:526–9.

17. Sandmire HF, O'Halloin TJ. Shoulder dystocia: its incidence and associated risk factors. *Int J Gynaecol Obstet* 1988;26:65–73.

18. Usha Kiran TS, Hemmadi S, Bethel J, Evans J. Outcome of pregnancy in a woman with an increased body mass index. *BJOG* 2005;112:768–72.

19. Royal College of Obstetricians and Gynaecologists. *Shoulder dystocia*. Green-top Guideline No. 42. London: RCOG; 2011 [http://www.rcog.org.uk/womens-health/clinical-guidance/shoulder-dystocia-green-top-42].

20. Lurie S, Ben-Arie A, Hagay Z. The ABC of shoulder dystocia management. *Asia Oceania J Obstet Gynaecol* 1994;20:195–7.

21. Hinshaw K. Shoulder dystocia. In: Johanson R, Cox C, Grady K, Howell C (editors). *Managing Obstetric Emergencies and Trauma. The MOET Course Manual*. London: RCOG Press; 2003:165–74.

22. Bruner JP, Drummond SB, Meenan AL, Gaskin IM. All-fours maneuver for reducing shoulder dystocia during labor. *J Reprod Med* 1998;43:439–43.

23. Sandberg EC. The Zavanelli maneuver: a potentially revolutionary method for the resolution of shoulder dystocia. *Am J Obstet Gynecol* 1985;152:479–84.

24. Vaithilingam N, Davies D. Cephalic replacement for shoulder dystocia: three cases. *BJOG* 2005;112:674–5.

25. Spellacy WN. The Zavanelli maneuver for fetal shoulder dystocia. Three cases with poor outcomes. *J Reprod Med* 1995;40:543–4.

26. Goodwin TM, Banks E, Millar LK, Phelan JP. Catastrophic shoulder dystocia and emergency symphysiotomy. *Am J Obstet Gynecol* 1997;177:463–4.

27. Gherman R. Posterior axillary sling traction: another empiric technique for shoulder dystocia alleviation? *Obstet Gynecol* 2009;113:478–9.

28. Hofmeyr GJ, Cluver CA. Posterior axilla sling traction for intractable shoulder dystocia. *BJOG* 2009;116:1818–20.

29. Maternal and Child Health Research Consortium. *Confidential Enquiry into Stillbirths and Deaths in Infancy: 5th Annual Report, 1 January–31 December 1996*. London: Maternal and Child Health Research Consortium; 1998.

30. Leung TY, Stuart O, Sahota DS, Suen SS, Lau TK, Lao TT. Head-to-body delivery interval and risk of fetal acidosis and hypoxic ischaemic encephalopathy in shoulder dystocia: a retrospective review. *BJOG* 2011;118:474–9.

31. Metaizeau JP, Gayet C, Plenat F. [Brachial plexus birth injuries. An experimental study (author's transl)]. *Chir Pediatr* 1979;20:159–63. Article in French.

32. MacKenzie IZ, Shah M, Lean K, Dutton S, Newdick H, Tucker DE. Management of shoulder dystocia: trends in incidence and maternal and neonatal morbidity. *Obstet Gynecol* 2007;110:1059–68.

Module 10
Cord prolapse

Key learning points

- To recognise the risk factors for cord prolapse.
- To call for appropriate help.
- To perform manoeuvres to reduce cord compression.
- To communicate effectively with the woman and the team.
- To understand the importance of appropriate documentation.

Common difficulties observed in training drills

- Recognition of occult cord prolapse.
- Inappropriate handling of the cord.
- Delay in moving woman to an appropriate position to relieve cord compression.
- Not calling for appropriate help.
- Difficulties with equipment for bladder filling.
- Omitting cord gases post-birth.

Introduction

Cord prolapse has been defined as the descent of the umbilical cord through the cervix, either alongside (occult) or past (overt) the presenting part, in the presence of ruptured membranes.

The incidence of umbilical cord prolapse ranges from 0.1% to 0.6% of all births.[1-3] In breech presentations it is around 1%.[4]

Risk factors for cord prolapse

Cord prolapse most commonly occurs after the amniotic membranes rupture (spontaneously or artificially) and the fetal presenting part is poorly applied to the maternal cervix. The umbilical cord slips below the presenting part and may subsequently be compressed, compromising the fetal blood supply.

The presence of risk factors (Box 10.1) should raise awareness, but the occurrence of cord prolapse remains extremely unpredictable. A common feature of all the risk factors is a poorly applied fetal presenting part.

Box 10.1 Risk factors for cord prolapse	
Antenatal	**Intrapartum**
Breech presentation	Amniotomy (especially with a high presenting part)
Unstable lie	
Oblique or transverse lie	Prematurity
Polyhydramnios	Breech presentation
External cephalic version	Internal podalic version
Expectant management of premature rupture of membranes	Second twin
	Disimpaction of fetal head during rotational assisted delivery
Previous cord prolapse	
	Fetal scalp electrode application

Prevention

The RCOG recommends that women with transverse, oblique or unstable lie should be offered elective admission to hospital at 37 weeks (or sooner if there are signs of labour or suspicion of ruptured membranes)[5] before elective caesarean section at term. Elective admission does not prevent cord prolapse; however, if cord prolapse does occur while in hospital, immediate diagnosis and treatment is possible, improving neonatal outcome.

If the cord is palpated below the presenting part on vaginal examination during labour, artificial rupture of membranes should be avoided.[5]

Any obstetric intervention after the membranes have ruptured (application of fetal scalp electrode, manual rotation of vertex, internal podalic version) carries a risk of cord prolapse, and upward displacement of the presenting part after membrane rupture should therefore be minimised.

Artificial rupture of the membranes should be avoided if the presenting part is unengaged and/or mobile. If artificial rupture of the membranes is absolutely necessary, it should be performed in, or near, the operating theatre with facilities to perform an immediate emergency caesarean section if required. In addition, fundal pressure and/or stabilisation of a longitudinal lie may reduce the risk of cord prolapse in these circumstances.

Perinatal complications

The maternal mortality rate associated with cord prolapse has fallen over the past century. However, the perinatal mortality rate associated with umbilical cord prolapse remains high (approximately 9%),[2] and cases of cord prolapse still consistently feature in perinatal mortality enquiries.

The interval between diagnosis and birth is significantly related to stillbirth and perinatal death. Cord prolapse outside hospital carries a significantly worse prognosis, and delays associated with transfer to hospital have been identified as a contributory factor when cord prolapse complicates home birth.[2,9–11]

Infants may suffer birth asphyxia owing to umbilical cord compression and/or arterial vasospasm of the umbilical cord secondary to exposure to vaginal fluids and/or air, which may result in hypoxic–ischaemic encephalopathy, cerebral palsy or neonatal death.[7] However, perinatal death after umbilical cord prolapse has been demonstrated to relate more to the complications of prematurity and low birth weight– the predisposing cause – rather than intrapartum asphyxia.[2,8]

Initial management of cord prolapse

An outline for the management of cord prolapse is shown in Figure 10.1. This is described in detail in the next section.

RECOGNISE – cord prolapse

Early diagnosis is important. A cord prolapse may be obvious when there is a loop of umbilical cord protruding through the vulva. However, a prolapsed cord is not always apparent and may only be found on vaginal examination.

Cord prolapse should be suspected when there is an abnormal fetal heart rate pattern (e.g. bradycardia, decelerations) in the presence of ruptured membranes, particularly if such changes commence soon after membrane

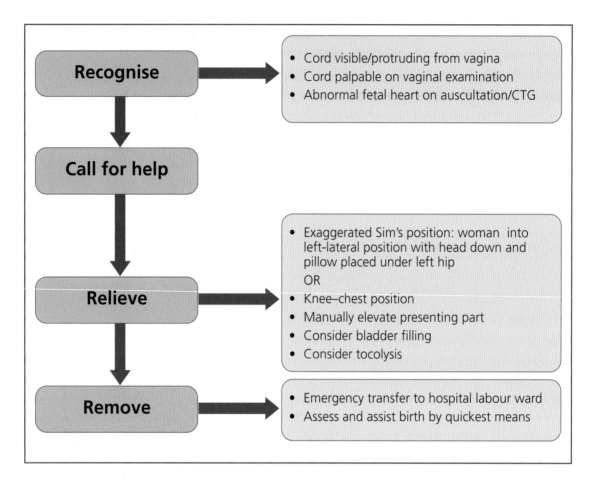

Figure 10.1 Outline of management of cord prolapse

rupture. A speculum and/or a digital vaginal examination should be performed when cord prolapse is suspected, regardless of gestation. Mismanagement of abnormal fetal heart rate patterns is one of the most common aspects of substandard care identified in perinatal death associated with cord prolapse.[5]

Call for help

As soon as cord prolapse is diagnosed, urgent help should be called immediately, including (if possible) a senior midwife, additional midwifery staff, the most experienced obstetrician available, an anaesthetist, the theatre team and the neonatal team.

If cord prolapse occurs outside hospital, an emergency ambulance should be called immediately to transfer the woman to the nearest obstetric unit. Even if birth appears imminent, a paramedic ambulance should still be called in case of neonatal compromise at birth.

When help arrives, 'cord prolapse' should be clearly stated so that all in attendance immediately understand the problem. Staff outside the obstetric unit (midwives, ambulance staff, general practitioners) should liaise directly with the obstetric unit, clearly stating that they are transferring a woman with a cord prolapse and giving an estimated time of arrival at hospital. This will ensure that the appropriate hospital staff are aware and preparations can be made to assist a timely birth upon arrival at hospital.

RELIEVE – cord compression

As soon as cord prolapse has been recognised, cord compression should be minimised by elevating the presenting part. This can be achieved by digital elevation of the presenting part, maternal positioning or bladder filling. Tocolysis may also be used to reduce uterine contractions.

Maternal positioning

Traditionally, management of umbilical cord prolapse has recommended the knee–chest face-down position. However, this position is less suitable for transportation and therefore the exaggerated Sim's position (left-lateral with a pillow under the left hip) with or without Trendelenburg (tilted bed so that the woman's head is lower than the pelvis) may be used instead (Figure 10.2).

Digital elevation of the presenting part

If cord prolapse is recognised at the time of rupture of membranes, the fingers should be kept within the vagina to elevate the presenting part. This reduces compression of the cord, particularly during contractions. If the umbilical cord has prolapsed out from the vagina, attempt to gently replace it back into the vagina with minimal handling.

There is no evidence to support the practice of covering the exposed cord with sterile gauze soaked in warmed saline.

Reduce contractions

If an oxytocin infusion is in progress, this should be stopped immediately.

Tocolysis has been used to reduce contractions and improve fetal bradycardia when there is a cord prolapse. Terbutaline 0.25 mg subcutaneously has been recommended.[12–14]

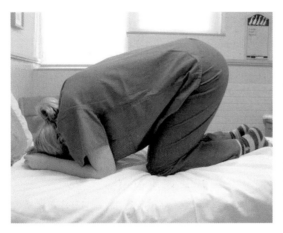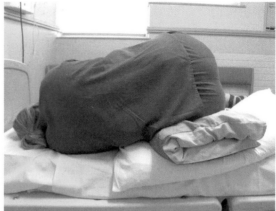

Figure 10.2 Maternal positioning to aid elevation of presenting part: (a) knee–chest; (b) exaggerated Sim's position

Bladder filling

If the decision-to-birth interval is likely to be prolonged, particularly if it involves ambulance transfer into hospital, elevation of the presenting part through bladder filling may be considered.

Bladder filling was first proposed by Vago in 1970[15] as a method of relieving pressure on the umbilical cord. Bladder filling raises the presenting part of the fetus off the compressed cord for an extended period of time, thereby eliminating the need for an examiner's fingers to displace the presenting part.[16]

A Foley catheter is placed into the urinary bladder. The bladder is filled via the catheter with sterile physiological (0.9%) saline using an intravenous blood infusion set. The catheter should be clamped once 500–750 ml has been instilled. It is essential to empty the bladder again just before any method of birth is attempted.

> **Any of the measures described above may be useful during preparation for assisting the birth of the fetus; however, birth should not be delayed by trying to implement these measures.**

Assessment of fetal wellbeing

Continuous electronic fetal monitoring should be performed. If there is no audible fetal heart, an ultrasound scan should be performed.

REMOVE – transport and assist birth

Cord prolapse should be managed in a unit with full anaesthetic and neonatal services. If cord prolapse occurs outside a labour ward, immediate transfer is essential.

Good communication is required so that appropriate members of staff are ready to receive the mother on arrival. Theatre should be on standby.

If there is no intravenous access, site a wide-bore intravenous cannula (14/16-gauge) and take blood for group and save and full blood count.

ASSESSMENT FOR BIRTH

- If the cervix is not fully dilated, caesarean section should be performed.
- If the cervix is fully dilated, consider an assisted vaginal birth as long as it is anticipated that it would be accomplished quickly and safely. Ventouse or forceps should be considered only if the prerequisites for operative birth are met.
- Breech extraction may be performed under some circumstances, for example after internal podalic version for the second twin.

In general, poor fetal outcomes are associated with more difficult attempts at achieving vaginal birth. It should be remembered that any delays could be compounded by the possible need to then undertake a caesarean section if an attempt at an instrumental birth fails.

The use of temporary measures, as described in the previous section, to relieve pressure on the cord should enable an attempt at regional anaesthesia (spinal or epidural top-up). However, prolonged and repeated attempts at regional anaesthesia must be avoided.

The presenting part should be kept elevated while anaesthesia is undertaken. Clear communication about the urgency and timing of birth is required between the obstetric, midwifery and anaesthetic teams to ensure the safest method of anaesthesia for both mother and fetus.

Neonatal resuscitation

An experienced neonatal team must be present at birth to ensure full cardiorespiratory support is given to the neonate, if required. Paired umbilical cord gases should be taken after birth to aid assessment of the neonatal condition.

Documentation

Documentation should include the time the cord prolapse occurred, the time help was called and arrived, methods used to alleviate cord compression, the time of the decision to assist the birth and method and the time of birth. A pro forma may aid documentation; an example is given in Figure 10.3.

Parents

Cord prolapse is a frightening experience for the parents. It is important to explain what is happening and to give the mother clear instructions. The parents will need support and debriefing. Clinicians should be encouraged to visit the parents the following day and subsequently, if required, to discuss events, answer any questions and address concerns.

Training

With regular training, the manoeuvres to relieve cord compression can be conducted efficiently without delaying birth. A retrospective study examined the effect of team rehearsals, and the introduction of regular training was associated with both more frequent actions to relieve cord compression and a shorter diagnosis-to-birth interval; crucially, it was also associated with consistently better neonatal outcomes.[17]

Key points

- Cord prolapse is a life-threatening situation for the baby.
- Once a cord prolapse is recognised:
  - ☐ relieve the pressure on the cord
  - ☐ move the mother to an appropriate place of birth
  - ☐ deliver the baby by the safest and most expedient means.
- Document your actions clearly and legibly.
- Discuss events with the parents.

PROMPT
PRactical Obstetric Multi-Professional Training

Name...
Date of Birth.................................
Hospital No...................................

Cord Prolapse Documentation pro forma

Please tick the relevant boxes

Senior Midwife called: Yes ☐   No ☐

Time called:.....................   Time arrived:.....................   Name:.............................

Senior Obstetrician called: Yes ☐   No ☐

Time called:.....................   Time arrived:.....................   Name:.............................

Grade of Obstetrician:...

Neonatologist called: Yes ☐   No ☐

Time called:.....................   Time arrived:.....................   Name:.............................

Diagnosed at home or hospital: Home ☐   Hospital ☐

Time of diagnosis:...................................

Cervical dilatation at diagnosis:............. cm

Procedures used in managing cord prolapse				
Elevating the presenting part manually	Yes	☐	No	☐
Filling the bladder	Yes	☐	No	☐
Left lateral, head tilt down / Knee-Chest position		(Please circle)		
Tocolysis with sc Terbutaline	Yes	☐	No	☐

Mode of birth		Mode of Anaesthesia	
Normal	☐	GA	☐
Forceps	☐	Spinal	☐
Ventouse	☐	Epidural	☐
C/S	☐		
Other	☐		

Diagnosis to birth interval:.......................minutes

Neonatal outcome		
Apgar Scores:	Weight:........................kg	
1 min:	**Cord PH**	**Base Excess**
5 mins:	Venous:	
10 mins:	Arterial:	

Admission to NICU:
Yes ☐   No ☐   Reason:...

AIMS form completed: Yes ☐

Known Risk Factors? Please state:...

	Follow – up appointment offered?
Mother debriefed Yes ☐ No ☐	

Signature:...   Print:...

Designation:.....................................   Date:...

Figure 10.3 Example of cord prolapse documentation pro forma

References

1. Critchlow CW, Leet TL, Benedetti TJ, Daling JR. Risk factors and infant outcomes associated with umbilical cord prolapse: a population-based case–control study among births in Washington State. *Am J Obstet Gynecol* 1994;170:613–8.

2. Murphy DJ, MacKenzie IZ. The mortality and morbidity associated with umbilical cord prolapse. *Br J Obstet Gynecol* 1995;102:826–30.

3. Lin MG. Umbilical cord prolapse. *Obstetrical & Gynecological Survey* 2006;61:269–77.

4. Panter KR, Hannah ME. Umbilical cord prolapse: so far so good? *Lancet* 1996;347:74.

5. Royal College of Obstetricians and Gynaecologists. *Management of cord prolapse*. Green-top Guideline (draft). London: RCOG; 2008.

6. Phelan JP, Boucher M, Mueller E, McCart D, Horenstein J, Clark S. The nonlaboring transverse lie. A management dilemma. *J Reprod Med* 1986;31:184–6.

7. MacLennan A. A template for defining a causal relation between acute intrapartum events and cerebral palsy: international consensus statement. *BMJ* 1999;319:1054–9.

8. Ylä-Outinen A, Heinonen PK, Tuimala R. Predisposing and risk factors of umbilical cord prolapse. *Acta Obstet Gynecol Scand* 1985;64:567–70.

9. Breech Presentation at Onset of Labour. Confidential Enquiries into Stillbirths and Deaths in Infancy. 7th Annual Report. London: Maternal and Child Health Consortium; 2000.

10. Beard RJ, Johnson DA. Fetal distress due to cord prolapse through a fenestration in a lower segment uterine scar. *J Obstet Gynaecol Br Commonw* 1972;79:763.

11. Johnson KC, Daviss BA. Outcomes of planned home births with certified professional midwives: large prospective study in North America. *BMJ* 2005;330:1416.

12. Gruese ME, Prickett SA. Nursing management of umbilical cord prolaspe. *J Obstet Gynecol Neonatal Nurs* 1993;22:311–5.

13. Katz Z, Shoham Z, Lancet M, Blickstein I, Mogilner BM, Zalel Y. Management of labor with umbilical cord prolapse: a 5-year study. *Obstet Gynecol* 1988;72:278–81.

14. Siassakos D, Fox R, Draycott TJ, for the Guidelines and Audit Committee of the Royal College of Obstetricians and Gynaecologists. Umbilical Cord Prolapse. Clinical Guideline Green-Top Guideline No.26. London: RCOG, 2008.

15. Vago T. Prolapse of the umbilical cord: a method of management. *Am J Obstet Gynecol* 1970;107:967–9.

16. Caspi E, Lotan Y, Schreyer P. Prolapse of the cord: reduction of perinatal mortality by bladder instillation and cesarean section. *Isr J Med Sci* 1983;19:541–5.

17. Siassakos D, Hasafa Z, Sibanda T, Fox R, Donald F, Winter C, et al. Retrospective cohort study of diagnosis–delivery interval with umbilical cord prolapse: the effect of team training. *BJOG* 2009;116:1089–96.

Module 11
Vaginal breech birth

Key learning points

- Ensure continuous electronic fetal monitoring in labour (to continue after decision to perform a caesarean section).
- Ensure full cervical dilatation before commencing pushing.
- Ensure a **'hands off'** approach as much as possible.
- Await visualisation of the breech at the perineum before encouraging active pushing.
- Avoid traction on the breech.
- Understand the manoeuvres that may be required to assist a breech birth.

Common difficulties observed in training drills

- Reluctance to allow the breech to descend without intervention.
- Premature commencement of assisted breech manoeuvres.
- Pressure on non-bony prominences during those manoeuvres.

Introduction

The incidence of breech presentation in the UK is 3–4% at term, although it is much higher earlier in pregnancy (for example, at 28 weeks of gestation 20% of babies are breech presentation).

Breech presentation is associated with a higher perinatal morbidity and mortality than cephalic presentation, particularly with vaginal birth: prematurity, congenital malformations, birth asphyxia and trauma are all more common with breech presentations.[1] These risk factors should inform antenatal, intrapartum and neonatal management.

Definition

Breech presentation is where the presenting part of the fetus is the buttocks or feet; the breech can be extended, flexed or footling (Figure 11.1).

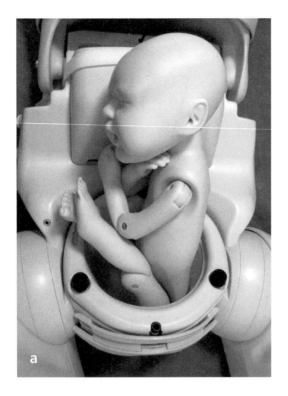

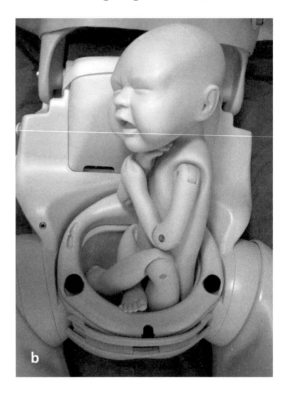

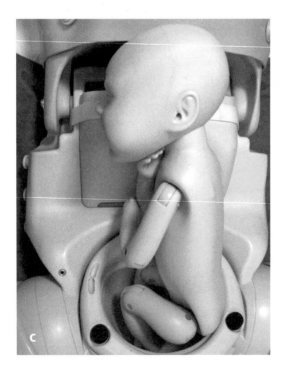

Figure 11.1 Types of breech presentation and incidence: (a) extended (65%): hips flexed, knees extended; (b) flexed (10%): hips flexed, knees flexed but feet not below the buttocks; (c) footling (25%): feet or knees are lowest (either single or double footling)

Predisposing factors

Factors that predispose to a breech presentation are listed in Box 11.1.

Box 11.1 Factors associated with breech presentation

Previous breech delivery	Uterine anomalies
Premature labour	Pelvic tumour or fibroids
High parity	Placenta praevia
Multiple pregnancy	Hydrocephaly/anencephaly
Polyhydramnios	Fetal neuromuscular disorders
Oligohydramnios	Fetal head and neck tumours

The rate of vaginal breech birth has declined over recent years from 1.2% in 1980 to 0.3% in 2001 and has continued to decline as a result of the Term Breech Trial.[2–4] This study compared outcomes after planned vaginal and planned caesarean births for breech presentation and demonstrated a significant reduction in perinatal morbidity and mortality in the planned caesarean group (reduction in mortality of 75%). In addition, there was no significant increase in maternal morbidity or mortality with planned caesarean births. However, the 2-year follow-up data from the trial have not demonstrated any statistically significant differences in neurodevelopment between the two groups. Therefore, it is unclear whether the long-term benefits for the child of planned caesarean section for breech presentation outweigh the maternal risks of the additional caesareans.

The optimal mode of birth for women in advanced labour or preterm labour with a breech presentation remains unclear and vaginal birth should be considered as an option in advanced labour, preterm birth and also for the second twin. For these reasons it is essential that practitioners maintain and practise their skills for assisted vaginal breech births. The RCOG recommendations for mode of birth are shown in Box 11.2.

Management of vaginal breech birth

Types of vaginal breech birth

Spontaneous breech birth: The fetus is allowed to deliver without assistance or manipulation. This accounts for a small proportion of deliveries, most of which are very preterm.

Assisted breech birth: The most common method of vaginal breech birth. The fetus is allowed to descend with the accoucheur employing a 'hands off' approach. However, recognised manoeuvres can be used to assist the birth as and when required.

Breech extraction: Mainly reserved for assisting the birth of the non-cephalic second twin. Breech extraction involves grasping one or both of the fetal feet from the uterine cavity and bringing them down through the vagina, before continuing with the manoeuvres used in an assisted breech birth. This should not be attempted in singleton pregnancies, as it is associated with a high rate of birth injury (25%) and mortality (10%).

Box 11.2 Summary of RCOG recommendations regarding mode of birth in breech presentation (adapted from RCOG Green-top Guideline No. 20b)[1]

- Neonatal morbidity and mortality is reduced by planned caesarean section in breech presentation at term.
- There is no evidence that caesarean section for the first or second twin (breech presentation) is beneficial.
- There is no evidence that caesarean section for a preterm breech is beneficial.
- There is no evidence that caesarean section for a labouring breech is beneficial.
- There is no evidence to support external cephalic version (ECV) for preterm breech.
- There is no evidence of long-term benefit in perinatal outcome for a breech presentation delivered by elective caesarean section.

Management of the first stage of labour

It is recommended that a vaginal breech birth should take place in a hospital with facilities for emergency caesarean section. There is no robust evidence available regarding the complications of breech birth outside the hospital setting.[1]

Preparation

Inform the senior midwife, senior obstetrician, anaesthetist and theatre staff of admission and ensure key members of staff are introduced to the parents.

Discuss the mode of birth again with the woman and ensure that she still wishes to opt for a vaginal breech birth. Discuss analgesia early in the process. There is no evidence to support routine epidural anaesthesia; there should be a range of analgesia offered during breech labour and birth.[1] Consider a pudendal block if there is no epidural analgesia.

Explain all delivery techniques and that a neonatologist will routinely attend a vaginal breech birth.

Establish intravenous access and take blood for full blood count and group and save.

The labour room and neonatal resuscitation equipment should be prepared. Ensure that prerequisites for an assisted vaginal breech birth are present: instrumental birth pack, forceps, lithotomy supports.

Electronic fetal monitoring

Continuous electronic fetal monitoring should be recommended to women with a breech presentation during labour and birth. The Seventh Annual report of the Confidential Enquiry into Stillbirth and Death in Infancy (CESDI) reviewed 56 deaths of singleton breech births and found clinical evidence of hypoxia before birth in all but one case.[2] The report concluded that: 'The assessments and decisions made by health professionals, during labour, in particular those regarding intrapartum fetal surveillance, were the critical factors in the avoidable deaths'.

A fetal scalp electrode can be placed on the fetal buttock if required, but fetal blood sampling is not recommended.[5]

Labour progress

Labour augmentation with oxytocin is not recommended. Amniotomy for labour augmentation should be performed with caution, but may be necessary for the use of internal fetal heart rate monitoring. Once spontaneous rupture of the membranes occurs, a vaginal examination should be performed to exclude a cord prolapse.

Management of the second stage of labour

If there is delay in the descent of the breech at any point in the second stage of labour, a caesarean section should be considered, as this may be a sign of relative fetopelvic disproportion.[1]

A breech birth should be attended by practitioners with adequate experience and skills to assist the birth, if required. The attendants should include a senior midwife, obstetrician and neonatologist (the senior midwife may also have valuable experience of vaginal breech births). An anaesthetist should be present on the labour ward at the time of birth and theatre staff should be on standby.

Women should be advised that, as most experience with vaginal breech birth is with the mother in the lithotomy position, this position should be routinely recommended for the actual birth; however, other positions have been described.[1] Once the breech is visible at the perineum, active pushing should be encouraged.

> **Remember: keep interventions to a minimum.**

Vaginal breech birth: assisted manoeuvres

- Episiotomy should be used selectively to facilitate birth.[1]
- Spontaneous birth of the limbs and trunk is preferable (Figure 11.2a), but the legs may need to be released by applying pressure to the popliteal fossae (Figure 11.2b).
- When handling the baby, it is important to ensure that support is provided over the bony prominences of the iliac crests to reduce the risk of soft-tissue internal injury.
- Ensure that the buttocks remain sacroanterior. Controlled rotation may be required if the trunk appears to be rotating to a sacroposterior position, but handling of the baby should be only over the bony prominences.

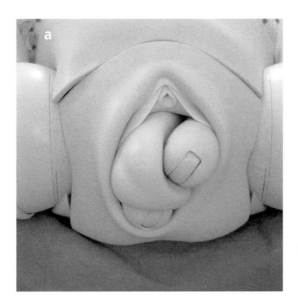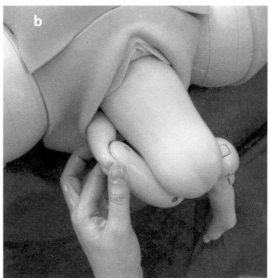

Figure 11.2 (a) Spontaneous birth of the limbs and trunk;
(b) applying pressure to the popliteal fossae

■ Avoid handling the umbilical cord as this increases vasospasm.

■ Encourage spontaneous birth until the scapulae are visible.

■ **Pulling on the infant's trunk can cause a nuchal arm and therefore should be avoided.**

■ If the arms are not released spontaneously, use the Løvsett's manoeuvre, as shown in Figure 11.3.

Engagement in the pelvis of the after-coming head

After release of the arms, support the baby until the nape of the neck becomes visible, using the weight of the baby to encourage flexion (Figure 11.4). If spontaneous birth of the head does not follow, an assistant may apply suprapubic pressure to assist flexion of the head.

Mauriceau–Smellie–Veit manoeuvre

The Mauriceau–Smellie–Veit manoeuvre may be required to assist birth of the aftercoming head (Figure 11.5). When using this manoeuvre, the baby's body should be supported on the flexor surface of the accoucheur's forearm. The first and third finger of the accoucheur's hand should be placed on the cheekbones (note that the middle finger is no longer placed in the fetal mouth as fetal injury has been reported). With the other hand, apply pressure to the occiput with the middle finger and place the other fingers

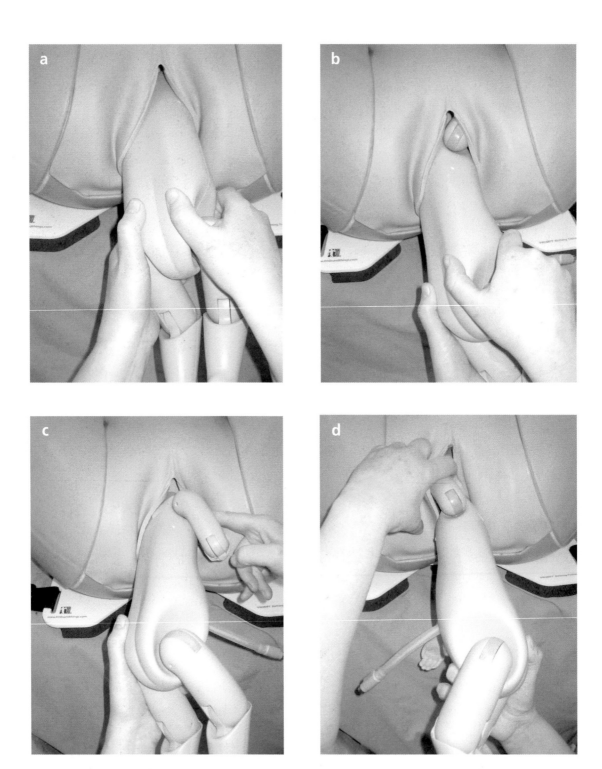

Figure 11.3 Løvsett's manoeuvre: (a) Gently hold the baby over the bony prominences of the hips and sacrum and rotate the baby so that one arm is uppermost (anterior); (b and c) to release the uppermost arm, an index figure should be placed over the baby's shoulder and follow the infant's arm to the antecubital fossa. The arm should be flexed for delivery; (d) following release of the first arm, rotate the baby 180 degrees, keeping the back uppermost, so that the second arm is now uppermost. Release this arm as described in (b).

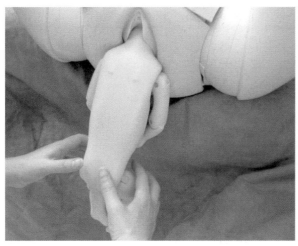 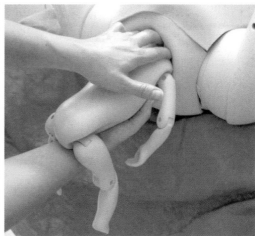

Figure 11.4 Nape of neck visible: using the weight of the baby to encourage flexion

Figure 11.5 The Mauriceau–Smellie–Veit manoeuvre for delivery of the aftercoming head

simultaneously on the fetal shoulders to promote flexion (i.e. keep the chin on the chest) (Figure 11.6).

Burns–Marshall technique

Another way of assisting the birth of the head is to raise the body vertically and have an assistant hold the baby's feet (Burns–Marshall technique). Sometimes, this will promote spontaneous birth of the head (Figure 11.7).

Forceps to assist birth of the head

Alternatively, the birth of the fetal head can be assisted with forceps. An assistant should hold the baby and the forceps should be applied from underneath the fetal body. The axis of traction should aim to flex the head (Figure 11.8). There is debate over which type of forceps should be used for this procedure and Kielland, Rhodes', Piper's and Wrigley's forceps have all been reported.

There is no experimental evidence to indicate which of the above techniques is preferable and previous experience of the practitioner may be an important factor in the decision as to which method is chosen. However, concern has been expressed about the risks of the Burns–Marshall method if used incorrectly, as it may lead to overextension of the baby's neck.[1]

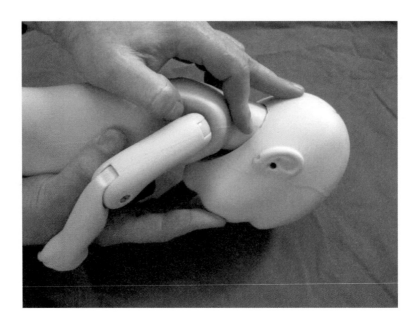

Figure 11.6 Flexion and birth of the fetal head using the Mauriceau–Smellie–Veit manoeuvre

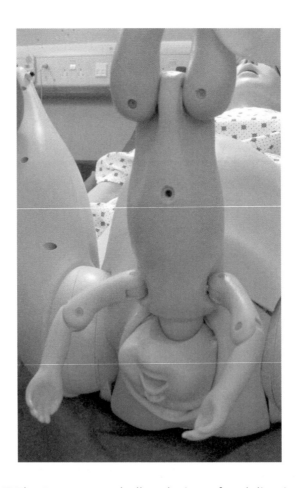

Figure 11.7 The Burns–Marshall technique for delivering the head

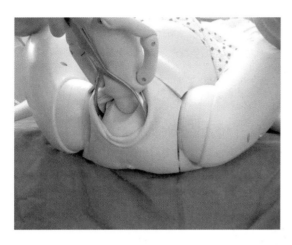 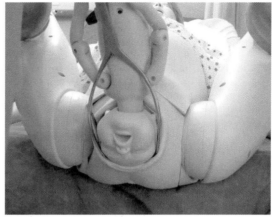

Figure 11.8 Kielland forceps to assist birth of the head

Complications and potential solutions

Failure to assist birth of the aftercoming head

If conservative methods and forceps fail to assist birth of the head, symphysiotomy or caesarean section should be performed. There have been successful births described by both symphysiotomy and rapid caesarean section when attempts to assist birth of the aftercoming head have failed.[1]

Head entrapment during a preterm breech delivery

The major cause of head entrapment is the passage of the preterm fetal trunk through an incompletely dilated cervix. In this situation, the cervix can be incised to release the head. The incisions should be made at the 10 and 2 o'clock positions, to avoid the cervical neurovascular bundles that run laterally in the cervix. Care should be taken as extension into the lower segment of the uterus can occur.[6]

Nuchal arms

This is when one or both of the arms become extended and trapped behind the fetal head. Nuchal arms complicate up to 5% of breech births (Figure 11.9) and may be caused by early traction on a breech. There is high morbidity associated with nuchal arms (25% risk of neonatal trauma, e.g. brachial plexus injuries) and therefore early traction on the breech should be avoided.

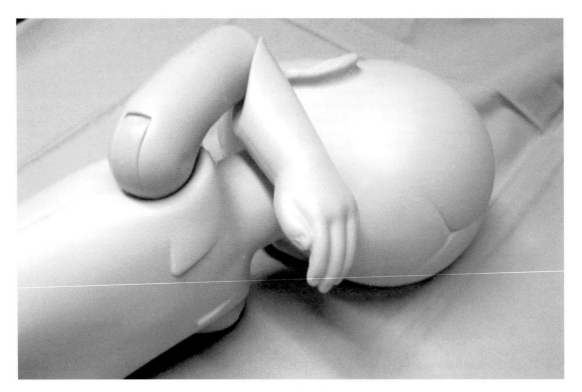

Figure 11.9 Nuchal arm

Nuchal arms can be released using Løvsett's manoeuvre and running the accoucheur's finger along the fetal arm to the antecubital fossa, applying pressure and flexing the arm for delivery.

Cord prolapse

Cord prolapse is more common with all breech presentations, especially footling breech presentations (10–25%). The most important factor with cord prolapse is prevention. Amniotomy should be undertaken with caution and with a presenting part filling the pelvis. The management of cord prolapse is outlined in **Module 10**.

Fetal risks associated with vaginal breech birth

Box 11.3 lists the risks associated with a vaginal breech birth. CESDI highlighted that the highest-risk group were undiagnosed breech presentations identified in labour.[2]

Box 11.3 Fetal risks associated with vaginal breech birth

Intrapartum death

Intracranial haemorrhage

Hypoxic ischaemic encephalopathy

Brachial plexus injury

Rupture of the liver, kidney or spleen

Dislocation of the neck, shoulder or hip

Fractured clavicle, humerus or femur

Cord prolapse

Occipital diastasis and cerebellar injury

References

1. Royal College of Obstetricians and Gynaecologists. *The management of breech presentation*. Green-top Guideline No. 20b. London: RCOG; 2006 [http://www.rcog.org.uk/womens-health/clinical-guidance/management-breech-presentation-green-top-20b].

2. Maternal and Child Health Research Consortium. *Confidential Enquiry into Stillbirths and Deaths in Infancy: 7th Annual Report, 1 January–31 December 1998*. London: Maternal and Child Health Research Consortium; 2000.

3. Department of Health (2002) NHS Maternity Statistics, England: 2001–02. Bulletin 2003/09 [www.dh.gov.uk/en/Publicationsandstatistics/Statistics/StatisticalWorkAreas/Statisticalhealthcare/DH_4086520].

4. Hannah ME, Hannah WJ, Hewson SA, Hodnett ED, Saigal S, Willan AR. Planned caesarean section versus planned vaginal birth for breech presentation at term: a randomised multicentre trial. Term Breech Trial Collaborative Group. *Lancet* 2002;356:1375–83.

5. National Collaborating Centre for Women's and Children's Health. *Intrapartum Care: care of healthy women and their babies during childbirth*. Clinical guideline. London: RCOG Press; 2007.

6. Robertson PA, Foran CM, Croughan-Minihane MS, Kilpatrick SJ. Head entrapment and neonatal outcome by mode of delivery in breech deliveries from 28 to 36 weeks of gestation. *Am J Obstet Gynecol* 1996;174:1742–7.

Further reading

James DK, Steer PJ, Weiner CP, Gonik B. *High Risk Pregnancy: Management Options*. 4th ed. London: Saunders; 2011.

Module 12
Twin birth

Key learning points

- Preparation of room and equipment for twin birth.
- Intrapartum electronic fetal monitoring of both twins.
- Stabilisation of the fetal lie of the second twin.
- To understand the various manoeuvres that facilitate birth of the second twin.
- Aim to keep twin–twin birth interval to less than 30 minutes.
- Justify situations in which caesarean section may be necessary.
- Recognise the risks of postpartum haemorrhage.
- Document details of birth accurately, clearly and legibly.

Common difficulties observed in training drills

- Not setting the room up with the necessary equipment prior to birth.
- Failure to maintain the stabilisation of the longitudinal fetal lie of the second twin until the presenting part has engaged into the pelvis.
- Premature amniotomy for the second twin.

Introduction

'Non-identical' (dizygotic) twins are the most common form of twins and result from fertilisation of two ova (eggs). Dizygotic twins are genetically no more similar than siblings, having separate placental circulations and gestational sacs (dizygotic, diamniotic, dichorionic).

'Identical' (monozygotic) twins are less common. They result from the splitting of a single developing embryo and are genetically identical. The degree of separation depends on the developmental stage at which the split takes place, and can be anything from separate circulations (monozygotic, monochorionic, diamniotic) to conjoined twins.[1]

The incidence of monozygotic twins is fairly constant. The rate of dizygotic twins varies considerably and there has recently been an increase owing to the use of fertility treatments and the increasing number of older mothers.[2] In England and Wales, the multiple maternity rate in 2010 was 15.7 multiple births per 1000 women giving birth compared with 9.6 in 1976.[3]

All twins share increased risks of preterm birth and fetal growth restriction, but monochorionic (identical) twin pregnancies have the added risk of twin-to-twin transfusion syndrome as they are dependent on a shared placenta and umbilical circulation. Around one-third of twin pregnancies in the UK have a monochorionic placenta.

The perinatal mortality rate of twins is seven-fold that of singletons and almost every obstetric complication is more common. Much of this excess perinatal mortality is attributable to antepartum factors; however, some of the mortality is related to problems during labour and at birth. Box 12.1 lists some of the risks of twin pregnancies both antenatally and in labour.

Box 12.1 Risks of twin pregnancies

Fetal growth restriction

Twin-to-twin transfusion (in monochorionic pregnancies)

Cord entanglement (monochorionic, monoamniotic)

Preterm labour (50% of twins deliver preterm)

Malpresentation

Cord prolapse

Neonatal seizures

Increased respiratory morbidity

Increased risk of cerebral palsy (four times the risk of a singleton pregnancy)

Postpartum haemorrhage for mother

As a consequence, twin pregnancies require specialist antenatal and intrapartum care in a consultant-led unit. The woman and her partner should be counselled regarding the mode and management of their twin birth prior to the onset of labour.

Presentation

Approximately 30% of twins present as cephalic/cephalic [4] (Figure 12.1), 35% of twins present as cephalic/non-cepahlic [4] (Figure 12.2), and the remaining 25% of twins present with the leading baby in a non-cephalic presentation at birth[4] (Figures 12.3 and 12.4).

Mode of birth

The optimal method of birth in twin pregnancies remains unclear. The Twin Birth Study aims to address this question.[5] It is an international multicentre randomised controlled trial comparing planned caesarean section with planned vaginal birth for twins at 32–38 weeks of gestation when the first twin is a vertex presentation. The primary outcome of the study is perinatal or neonatal mortality and/or serious neonatal morbidity.[5]

Vaginal birth of the second twin is recognised as a time of high risk. A recent retrospective review of twin births in England, Northern Ireland and Wales between 1994 and 2003 concluded that, at term, the second twin had a greater than two-fold higher risk of perinatal death related to birth and a greater than three-fold higher risk of death caused by intrapartum anoxia.[6]

The planned mode of birth is dependent on presentation, amnionicity and chorionicity, predicted fetal weight, gestation and fetal and maternal wellbeing.[1]

In otherwise uncomplicated twin pregnancies at term where the first twin is cephalic, a vaginal birth should be offered (assuming there are no other relative or absolute contraindications to vaginal birth). However, it is important to emphasise to the mother that serious acute intrapartum problems following the birth of the first twin (for example conversion to transverse lie, cord prolapse, prolonged time interval to birth of the second twin) which may lead to emergency caesarean section, perinatal death and neonatal morbidity can occur even in cephalic/cephalic presentations.

When the first twin is not cephalic, an elective caesarean section should be offered. This recommendation has been reinforced by the findings of the Term Breech Trial, which showed increased morbidity and mortality with vaginal breech birth in singleton pregnancies.[7]

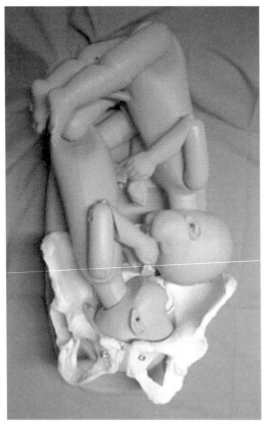

Figure 12.1 Cephalic, cephalic

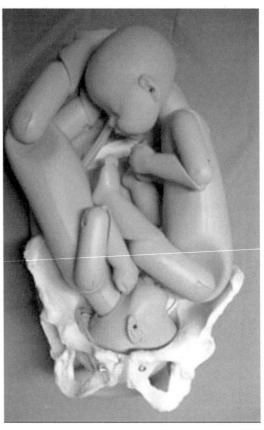

Figure 12.2 Cephalic, breech

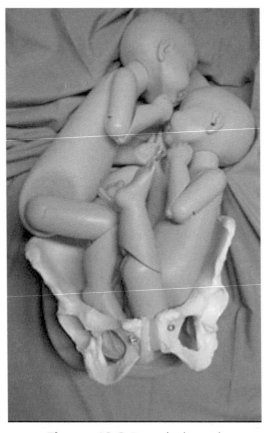

Figure 12.3 Breech, breech

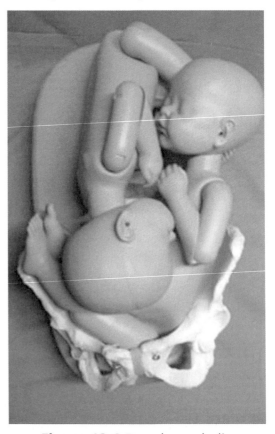

Figure 12.4 Breech, cephalic

It is widely accepted that the birth of monoamniotic and conjoined twins should be by elective caesarean section.[8]

Timing of birth

The majority of women with a twin pregnancy will labour spontaneously by 37 weeks of gestation. There is no robust evidence to indicate the optimal timing of birth in either identical/monochorionic or non-identical/dichorionic twin pregnancies, but the incidence of stillbirth in twins after 37–38 weeks of gestation is higher than in singleton pregnancies.[9] The RCOG recommends that delivery should be planned at 37–38 weeks of gestation in otherwise uncomplicated dichorionic twin pregnancies and at 36–37 weeks of gestation in otherwise uncomplicated monochorionic twin pregnancies.[10]

Management of vaginal twin birth

All women should have a discussion in the antenatal period with a midwife and a senior obstetrician about their planned intrapartum care. These discussions should be documented in the relevant part of the women's handheld notes.

The discussion should explain:

- that there is an increased risk of morbidity for the second twin
- analgesia, including the advantages and disadvantages of epidural anaesthesia
- the possibility of presumed fetal compromise in the second twin
- stabilisation of the fetal lie
- the use of oxytocin to augment contractions in the inter-twin period
- the possibility of intervention to expedite birth of the second twin
- that there is a small risk of caesarean section even after successful vaginal birth of the first twin
- active management of the third stage of labour and the use of an oxytocin infusion to reduce the risk of postpartum haemorrhage.

First stage of labour

All women with a multiple pregnancy who are in labour should be given one-to-one care by an experienced midwife and should be reviewed by the most senior obstetrician available. The anaesthetist and neonatologist and neonatal care unit should be informed of the mother's admission. The midwife and obstetrician should discuss the woman's birth plan with the woman and her birthing partner. A clear plan should be documented in the notes. An example of an admission checklist is given in Figure 12.4.

Fetal blood sampling of the first twin may be performed if indicated. If there are concerns for the wellbeing of the second twin, a caesarean section is indicated as a fetal blood sample cannot be performed.

	Tick when completed	Comments
Introduce the parents to the team.		
Review the handheld and hospital notes including the care plan to identify any antenatal risk factors.		
Explain the plan for birth.		
Establish intravenous access, take blood for full blood count (FBC) and group and save (G&S).		
Confirm presentation of both twins with ultrasound.		
Continuous electronic fetal monitoring is recommended: • A scalp electrode may be used for twin I to help differentiate the fetal heart recordings. • Ultrasound can be used to identify the optimal location placement of the EFM transducers. • A suitable monitor should be used to enable the differentiation of the two fetal heart tracings.		
Discuss analgesia. An epidural is helpful as it will make any intrauterine manipulation of twin II easier and can be used for caesarean section if needed.		
Consider giving ranitidine 150 mg PO every 6 hours.		
Obstetrician to document a care plan for twin birth in the handheld record.		
Date: Name: Signature: Grade:		

Figure 12.4 An example of a checklist on admission to labour ward

Oxytocin augmentation is not contraindicated for hypotonic contractions in labour but should be discussed with a senior obstetrician.

Second stage of labour

A twin birth should be supervised by an experienced obstetrician. Healthcare professionals attending the birth should include:

- at least two midwives (preferably experienced)
- at least one experienced obstetrician
- at least two members of the neonatal team
- an anaesthetist and operating department practitioner (available on the labour ward).

Prepare the labour room and required healthcare staff in advance so that there is a calm and unhurried approach to the birth.

Prepare the room and staff

Ensure prerequisites for twin birth are present. A local checklist may be helpful. A list of the equipment required is shown in Box 12.1.

An oxytocin infusion should be prepared and ready to be commenced after the birth of the first twin as contractions sometimes stop or reduce in frequency at this stage.

Prepare the mother

Keep the mother informed. Explain who will be present at the twin birth and also their roles.

Twin birth – procedure

The birth of the first twin is performed as for a singleton birth. The midwife who is caring for the mother can assist the birth of the first twin (and the second twin) if there are no problems.

After the first twin is born, an assistant (preferably an experienced obstetrician) should stabilise the lie of the second twin until the presenting part descends into the pelvis. This is achieved by the assistant placing both hands on the mother's abdomen and holding the fetus in a longitudinal axis. The presentation of the second twin and also the optimal place to monitor its heart rate should be identified by ultrasound scan.

Box 12.1 Equipment required for a twin birth

Ultrasound scanner

Lithotomy set (if in theatre)

Operative birth trolley

Forceps and ventouse (silastic and kiwi)

Twin pack (two sets of cord clamps)

Four cord blood sampling syringes

Two resuscitaires

Two sets of baby linen and hats

Oxytocin infusion 3 units in 50 ml normal saline (ready to be commenced after birth of the first twin)

Syntocinon or Syntometriene for third stage of labour as appropriate

Oxytocin infusion 40 units and 500 ml normal saline (for prophylactic use after third stage of labour) – ready to be made up and administered after birth of both twins, but kept separate from oxytocin infusion used between first and second twin

---

There should be continuous CTG monitoring of the second twin after the birth of the first twin. If there are any CTG abnormalities, the birth of the second twin must be expedited.

The uterine contractions may stop or become irregular. Therefore, be prepared to commence an oxytocin infusion soon after the birth of the first twin; for example, oxytocin infusion 3 units in 50 ml normal saline started at a rate of 4 mu/minute (4 ml/hour) with the rate doubled every 5 minutes until regular contractions return, to a maximum infusion rate of 20 mu/minute (20 ml/hour). Oxytocin should only be commenced once the lie of the second twin has been confirmed as longitudinal.

If the lie is longitudinal, await descent of the presenting part so that it is low in the pelvis before performing an amniotomy.

With regular contractions the presenting part will descend and, once it becomes fixed in the pelvis, artificial rupture of the membranes can then be performed during a contraction.

Provided the CTG is normal, expectant management is advisable, allowing natural progress to a vaginal birth (either cephalic or breech).

The aim should be for the second twin to be born within 30 minutes of the first twin. However, if there is delay and an assisted birth is required, as long as the CTG is normal it may still be better to wait for spontaneous descent of the presenting part before performing artificial rupture of the membranes and intervening to assist the birth.

If there is delay or evidence of fetal compromise, an assisted birth is indicated.

If the lie of the second twin is transverse, there are two options:

- external cephalic version
- internal podalic version.

External cephalic version

When attempting external cephalic version (Figure 12.5), the ultrasound probe can be used as a 'hand' so that fetal lie and heart rate can be monitored throughout.

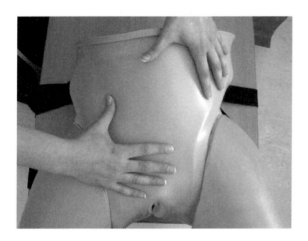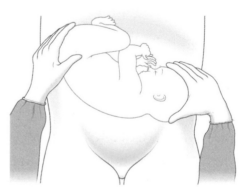

Figure 12.5 External cephalic version

Internal podalic version

With internal podalic version, one or both fetal feet are grasped inside the uterus before proceeding to a breech extraction (Figure 12.6). Before any traction is applied, the operator must confirm that they are holding a foot by

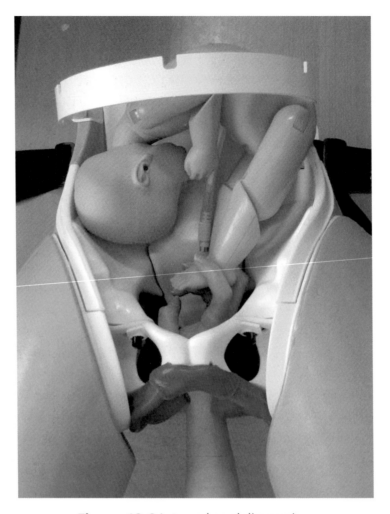

Figure 12.6 Internal podalic version

feeling the heel. It is important to try not to rupture the membranes too early, in order to avoid cord prolapse.

The same manoeuvres used for an assisted breech birth may be needed to assist birth of the second twin. Remember that twins are likely to be smaller than singleton fetuses. In cases of preterm twins, the cervix can close around the head of a breech baby. Note that sometimes the second twin may be considerably bigger than the first twin, and this too can cause problems during birth. Therefore, it is useful to check the estimated fetal weights from the last routine ultrasound scan.

Several studies have reviewed outcomes after external cephalic version compared with internal podalic version, and have concluded that there were no differences in neonatal or maternal outcomes. However, internal podalic version followed by breech extraction was associated with a higher rate of success of vaginal birth and lower caesarean section rates.

The length of inter-twin birth interval

The length of the inter-twin birth interval is variable. Although a longer inter-twin birth interval is associated with a continuous slow decline in umbilical cord pH, the small differences in pH between 15 and 30 minutes were not large enough to impact on clinical management.[11] However, it is widely accepted that the interval should ideally be no longer than 30 minutes.

There are theoretical concerns regarding the risk of acute inter-fetal transfusion in monochorionic twins following the birth of the first twin. These risks have not been substantiated; however, it would be prudent to clamp the cord of the first twin as soon as possible after its birth.[10]

Third stage of labour

Double-clamp the umbilical cord following each birth and place an additional cord clamp on the placental end of the cord of the second twin so it can be identified after delivery.

Paired umbilical cord gas bloods should be taken from the cords of both twins.

Owing to the high risk of postpartum haemorrhage, a bolus of oxytocin should be given immediately after the birth of the second twin. An oxytocin infusion should then be commenced and run according to local protocol. It is very important to continue to observe the mother for signs of postpartum haemorrhage.

As with all complicated births, careful and precise documentation is paramount. Figure 12.7 is an example of a documentation pro forma that may be used to record a twin birth.

Name:	Hospital Number:		Date:
Gestation:			Comments:
Chorionicity	Dichorionic/diamniotic or Monochorionic/diamniotic		
	Twin I	**Twin II**	
Presentation at start of 2nd stage	Cephalic Breech Other	Cephalic Breech Other	
CTG	Normal Suspicious Pathological	Normal Suspicious Pathological	
Syntocinon infusion	Yes No	Yes No	
Analgesia	None Entonox Epidural Spinal GA	None Entonox Epidural Spinal GA	
IV access	Yes No If no, reason for no access:		
Ranitidine	Yes: oral IV No		
Senior midwife present	Yes Name: No		
Obstetric registrar (ST3–5) present	Yes Name: No		
Senior obstetric registrar (ST6–7)	Yes Name: No		
Consultant obstetrician present	Yes Name: No		
Experienced neonatologist present at birth	Yes Name: No		
Mode of birth twin I Time:	Spontaneous vaginal Ventouse Forceps LSCS		
Syntocinon infusion between twins	Yes No		
Mode of birth twin II Time:	Spontaneous vaginal Ventouse Forceps LSCS Assisted breech Breech extraction		
	Twin I	**Twin II**	
Presentation at birth	Cephalic Breech Other	Cephalic Breech Other	
Internal or external manoeuvres performed	Yes: No	Yes: No	
Cord gases taken	Yes No	Yes No	
Apgars (at 1, 5, 10 minutes)			
Date: Name:	Signature:		Grade:

Figure 12.7 Example of a documentation pro forma to record a twin birth

References

1. Hofmeyr GJ, Barrett JF, Crowther CA. Planned caesarean section for women with a twin pregnancy. *Cochrane Database Syst Rev* 2011;(12):CD006553.

2. Australian Institute of Health and Welfare. *Australia's mothers and babies 2008*. Perinatal Statistics Series No. 24. Canberra: AIHW; 2010.

3. Office for National Statistics. Characteristics of Birth 2, England and Wales, 2010. London: Office for National Statistics; 2011.

4. Grisaru D, Fuchs S, Kuperminc MJ, Har-Toov J, Niv J, Lessing JB. Outcome of 306 twin deliveries according to first twin presentation and method of delivery. *Am J Perinatol* 2000;17:303–7.

5. The Twin Birth Study: planned caesarean section versus planned vaginal birth for twins at 32–38 weeks gestation

6. Smith GC, Fleming KM, White IR. Birth order of twins and risk of perinatal death related to delivery in England, Northern Ireland, and Wales, 1994–2003: retrospective cohort study. *BMJ* 2007;334:576.

7. Hannah ME, Hannah WJ, Hewson SA, Hodnett ED, Saigal S, Willan AR. Planned caesarean section versus planned vaginal birth for breech presentation at term: a randomised multicentre trial. Term Breech Trial Collaborative Group. *Lancet* 2000;356:1375–83.

8. Tessen JA, Zlatnik FJ. Monoamniotic twins: a retrospective controlled study. *Obstet Gynecol* 1991;77:832–4.

9. Hartley RS, Emanuel I, Hitti J. Perinatal mortality and neonatal morbidity rates among twin pairs at different gestational ages: optimal delivery timing at 37 to 38 weeks' gestation. *Am J Obstet Gynecol* 2001;184:451–8.

10. Royal College of Obstetricians and Gynaecologists. Management of monochorionic twin pregnancy. Green-top Guideline No. 51. London: RCOG; 2008 [http://www.rcog.org.uk/womens-health/clinical-guidance/management-monochorionic-twin-pregnancy].

11. McGrail CD, Bryant DR. Intertwin time interval: how it affects the immediate neonatal outcome of the second twin. *Am J Obstet Gynecol* 2005;192:1420–2.

Module 13
Acute uterine inversion

Key learning points

■ To recognise an inverted uterus and the accompanying maternal shock.

■ To summon appropriate help and ensure immediate management of maternal shock.

■ To outline mechanical manoeuvres to replace the uterus, including manually replacing the uterus as soon as possible.

■ To emphasise that the placenta should not be removed, if adherent, until the uterus has been replaced.

Common difficulties observed in training drills

■ Delay in recognition of the problem.

■ Not stating the problem clearly to those first attending the emergency call.

■ Delay in commencing resuscitation.

■ Delay in manually replacing the uterus.

■ Not being prepared for a subsequent postpartum haemorrhage

Introduction

Acute inversion of the uterus is a rare complication of childbirth. Incidence varies widely from as many as 1/1500 births to as few as 1/20 000 births.[1,2] There are no randomised controlled studies that have addressed the best management options, although some case reports recommend immediate replacement of the uterus as the most successful management strategy.[2]

Definition

When the uterus inverts, the fundus of the uterus descends abnormally through the genital tract, thus turning itself inside out. There are three grades of uterine inversion:

- grade I: fundus inverts down to the cervical canal
- grade II: fundus inverts into the vagina
- grade III: fundus is visible at the introitus.

There are several recognised risk factors for acute uterine inversion, as described in Box 13.1.[3,4]

Box 13.1 Risk factors for uterine inversion

Excessive traction on the umbilical cord

Inappropriate fundal pressure

Short umbilical cord

Multiparity

Abnormally adherent placenta

Vaginal birth after caesarean (VBAC)

Abnormalities of the uterus (e.g. unicornuate uterus)

Previous uterine inversion

Fetal macrosomia

Precipitate labour

Connective tissue disorders (e.g. Marfan syndrome, Ehlers–Danlos syndrome)

Diagnosis

Uterine inversion can be difficult to diagnose, particularly if the fundus is not outside the introitus. The development of sudden maternal shock is most commonly the first sign of a uterine inversion, and is frequently unexpected as there is often minimal blood loss.

An abdominal and vaginal examination should be performed early. Grade III uterine inversion is characterised by a mass (uterus) protruding through the introitus (Figure 13.1). However, there should be a high index of suspicion

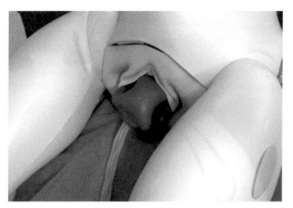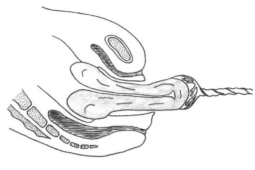

Figure 13.1 A grade III uterine inversion

for uterine inversion when the uterine fundus is not palpable on abdominal examination.

As the uterus inverts through the cervix, it stimulates the vagus nerve, leading to vasovagal (neurogenic) shock, which is characterised by bradycardia[3] and hypotension.[4]

Clinically, the woman often looks as if she has fainted, but there is minimal blood loss. However, hypovolaemic shock with tachycardia and hypotension may also occur if a postpartum haemorrhage follows the uterine inversion. All women should be treated with standard initial resuscitation; however, the quickest way to resolve neurogenic shock is to return the uterus to its anatomical position.[3]

> **Uterine inversion is associated with atonic postpartum haemorrhage in over 90% of cases.[3,5] This occurs once the uterus has been replaced and the placenta has been removed. Care should be taken to accurately measure blood loss as this is often underestimated.[6]**

Management

Immediate action

Figure 13.2 provides an algorithm for immediate management of an inverted uterus.

The treatment of maternal shock should be addressed immediately and appropriate assistance should be called.

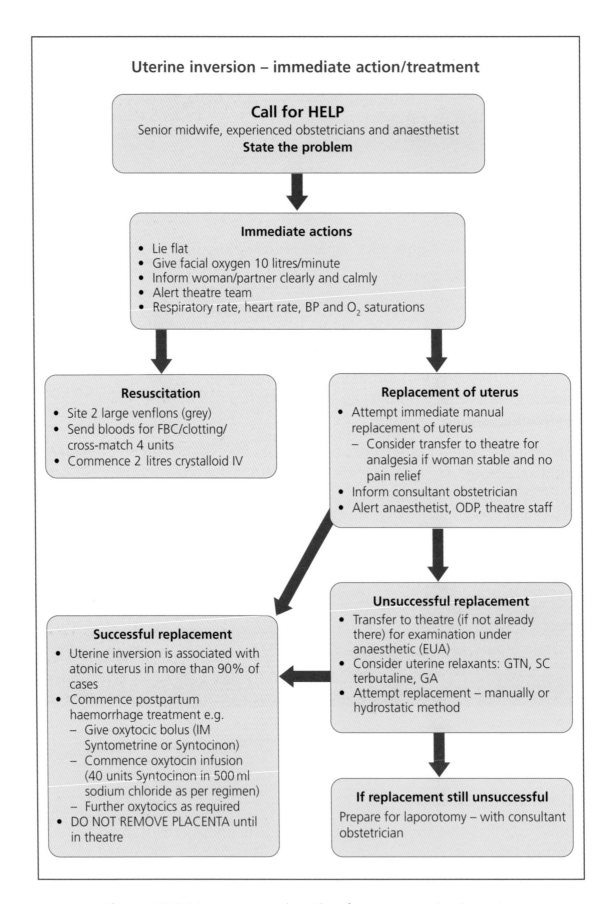

Figure 13.2 Management algorithm for acute uterine inversion

- Call for help: this should include a senior midwife, the most experienced obstetrician available and an anaesthetist.
- Give high-flow oxygen (10 l/minute) via a facemask with reservoir.
- Clearly and calmly inform the woman of the need to immediately reposition the uterine fundus.
- Treatment of the uterine inversion and resuscitation should take place simultaneously:

Resuscitation

- Site two large-bore intravenous cannulae.
- Commence intravenous infusion of 2 litres of Hartmann's solution.
- Take blood and send for cross-match (4 units), full blood count and clotting. (The main complication associated with uterine inversion is atonic postpartum haemorrhage.[7])
- The quickest way to treat neurogenic shock is to replace the uterus.

Treatment

- The uterus should be replaced as soon as possible.
- If the woman is bleeding heavily, is haemodynamically unstable or already has effective analgesia, the accoucheur should manually replace the uterus immediately in the labour room or at home.
- If the woman is stable and does not have adequate analgesia, prompt transfer to theatre for analgesia should be considered prior to replacement.
- If replacement is successful, administer an intramuscular oxytocic bolus. This should be followed by an intravenous infusion of 40 units of oxytocin in 500 ml normal saline, administered over 4 hours.
- If replacement is unsuccessful, transfer the patient to the operating theatre.
- If a uterine inversion occurs outside the hospital:
  - ☐ Immediate replacement should be attempted and an emergency ambulance should be called.
  - ☐ If the uterus is successfully replaced, an oxytoxic should be administered and the woman should still be transferred to hospital.
  - ☐ If the uterus is not replaced, the woman should be transferred to the nearest obstetric unit as quickly as possible. The hospital should be informed so that the theatre team are ready on the woman's arrival.

Management of the inversion

The uterus can be manually replaced by putting a hand into the vagina and following the cord to the fundus; while supporting the inverted fundus in the palm of the hand, gently raise the uterus into the abdominal cavity and 'replace' it back to its anatomical position (Figure 13.3). If the placenta is still adherent, it should not be removed before uterine replacement.[2]

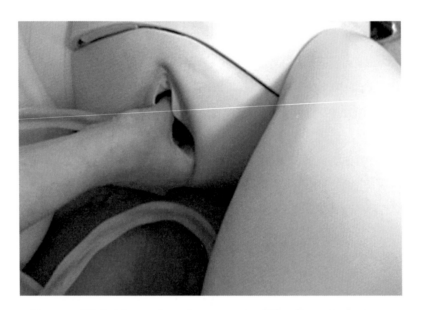

Figure 13.3 Manual replacement of the inverted uterus

The earlier the replacement of the uterus is attempted, the more likely it is to be successful.[5] As the uterus remains prolapsed it becomes more oedematous and a constriction ring may develop, making replacement more difficult.[3]

Uterine relaxants

Tocolysis can be useful to relax the uterus to assist manual correction of the inversion, particularly if a constriction ring has developed. Terbutaline (0.25 mg subcutaneously) or glyceryl trinitrate spray (one metered dose sublingually) can be used for this purpose. General anaesthesia may also promote uterine relaxation and can be useful if repeat attempts at uterine replacement are necessary.

> **Caution should be taken with the use of uterine relaxants as their use will exacerbate atonic postpartum haemorrhage once the uterus is replaced.**

Hydrostatic method for the management of an inverted uterus

Uterine inversion can be corrected using hydrostatic pressure to distend the vagina and push the fundus upward into its anatomical position. This technique was originally described by simply sealing the vaginal entrance with an assistant's hand;[8] however, a silastic ventouse cup can be used to create a better seal, thus improving the hydrostatic pressure (Figure 13.4).[9]

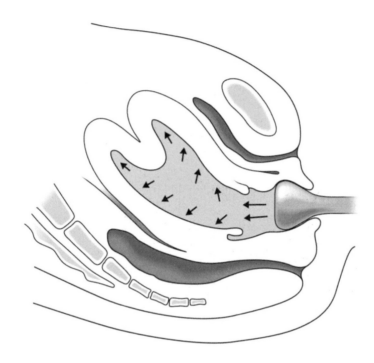

Figure 13.4 Hydrostatic method for the management of an inverted uterus

Equipment required:

■ silastic vacuum cup
■ blood-giving set
■ 2 litres of slightly warmed normal saline intravenous solution.

The silastic vacuum cup is placed within the vagina to occlude the vaginal opening. Two litres of slightly warmed intravenous normal saline (place the sealed saline bags in a bowl of warm water before infusing, if time allows) are rapidly infused through a blood-giving set which is attached directly to the end of the silastic vacuum cup. The fluid bag should be placed 100–150 cm above the level of the vagina to provide sufficient pressure for insufflation. Reduction of the inversion is usually achieved within 5–10 minutes of commencing this technique.

Continuing management

Once the uterus is successfully replaced, it should be manually held in position for a few minutes to promote uterine contraction and prevent re-inversion.[3] The use of an SOS Bakri tamponade balloon catheter (Cook® Medical Incorporated, Bloomington, IN, USA) has been described following replacement of the uterus to maintain the uterine position and prevent re-inversion, while concurrently assisting in the treatment of atony.[10] Oxytocics should be administered at this stage, with an initial bolus dose and an infusion over 4 hours, in view of the risk of postpartum haemorrhage.

> **If the placenta is adherent, it should be manually removed after the uterus has been replaced.**

Antibiotics should be administered in view of the infection risk with manual uterine replacement. Intravenous co-amoxiclav or similar broad-spectrum antibiotics should be given at the time of the procedure and may be continued for 24 hours, in line with local guidance and the woman's allergies.

Surgical management

In rare circumstances when the above techniques are unsuccessful, laparotomy may be required. Upward traction on the uterus from the abdominal cavity is used to achieve replacement to the anatomical position (Huntington's operation). If this procedure is unsuccessful, Haultain's operation, which involves vertically incising the cervical ring posteriorly to aid replacement of the uterus, can be performed.[3]

Documentation

It is important that all personnel involved and treatment administered are documented in the maternal notes as soon after the event as possible.

Debriefing after the emergency

Once the woman's clinical condition is stable and she is comfortable, she needs to be debriefed about the sudden event. This is best undertaken by one of the members of the team that managed the clinical problem. The woman may need to be told that:

■ it is difficult to predict recurrence, as experience with uterine inversion is limited

- hospital birth and active management of the third stage of labour is recommended for future pregnancies
- uterine inversion can occur outside pregnancy and childbirth.

References

1. Hussain M, Jabeen T, Liaquat N, Noorani K, Bhutta SZ. Acute puerperal uterine inversion. *J Coll Physicians Surg Pak* 2004;14:215–7.

2. Milenkovic M, Kahn J. Inversion of the uterus: a serious complication at childbirth. *Acta Obstet Gynecol Scand* 2005;84:95–6.

3. Bhalla R, Wuntakal R, Odejinmi F, Khan RU. Acute inversion of the uterus. *The Obstetrician & Gynaecologist* 2009;11:13–8.

4. Belfort M, Dildy G. Postpartum haemorrhage and other problems of the third stage. In: James DK, Steer PJ, Weiner CP, Gonik B (editors). *High Risk Pregnancy: Management Options*. 4ed. London: Saunders; 2011.

5. Watson P, Besch N, Bowes WA Jr. Management of acute and subacute puerperal inversion of the uterus. *Obstet Gynecol* 1980;55:12–6.

6. Beringer RM, Patteril M. Puerperal uterine inversion and shock. *Br J Anaesth* 2004;92:439–41.

7. Baskett TF. Acute uterine inversion: a review of 40 cases. *J Obstet Gynaecol Can* 2002;24:953–6.

8. O'Sullivan JV. Acute inversion of the uterus. *Br Med J* 1945;2:282–3.

9. Ogueh O, Ayida G. Acute uterine inversion: a new technique of hydrostatic replacement. *Br J Obstet Gynaecol* 1997;104:951–2.

10. Soleymani Majd S, Pilsniak A, Reginald PW. Recurrent uterine inversion: a novel treatment approach using SOS Bakri balloon. *BJOG* 2009;116:999–1001.

Module 14
Basic newborn resuscitation

Key learning points

■ To develop and practise a structured approach to the skills required in neonatal resuscitation.

■ To understand the causes of respiratory and cardiac arrest in the neonate and anticipate problems attributable to maternal obstetric history.

■ To understand the importance of calling for help early.

■ To communicate effectively to the parents and the neonatal team.

■ To complete accurate documentation.

Difficulties observed in previous neonatal resuscitation drills

■ Poor thermal care during resuscitation, especially in preterm infants.

■ Failure to open the infant's airway adequately, usually owing to over-extension of the neck.

■ Loss of effective airway maintenance, particularly when conducting simultaneous cardiac compressions.

■ Performing chest compressions too slowly.

Introduction

This module provides an outline of the process of basic newborn resuscitation but is not intended to be a complete guide. Further information is available from the Resuscitation Council (UK) publication *Newborn Life Support*.[1]

Background

All neonates experience a degree of hypoxia during the process of labour and birth, with respiratory exchange being interrupted for as long as 50–75 seconds with each contraction throughout labour. While most healthy babies tolerate this well, some do not and may require additional help to establish normal breathing once born.[1,2]

The fetus is designed to undertake the stress of labour and the neonate's brain can withstand much longer periods without oxygen than an adult brain. In addition, a neonate's heart can continue to beat effectively for 20 minutes or more without lung aeration, even after the reserve system of gasping has ceased. Therefore, the primary aim of newborn resuscitation is inflation of the lungs with air or oxygen, so that the still functioning circulation can then pump oxygenated blood to and from the heart to initiate recovery.[1,2]

Physiology of neonatal hypoxia

There are two centres in the brain that are responsible for the control of respiration; one is a higher centre.

If the hypoxic insult to the infant is sufficient, the fetus's breathing movements in utero become deeper and more rapid and eventually cease, as the centres responsible for controlling them are unable to function owing to lack of oxygen. This is known as the 'primary apnoea' phase.[2]

Once the fetus enters 'primary apnoea', the heart rate falls to about half its usual rate as the heart muscle switches from using aerobic to the less efficient anaerobic metabolism. Lactic acid build-up from anaerobic metabolism causes the fetus to become acidotic and the circulation is diverted away from non-essential organs.

After a variable length of time of continuing hypoxia, unconscious gasping activity is initiated. The fetus produces a shuddering, whole-body gasp at an approximate rate of 12 breaths/minute.[3] If these gasps fail to aerate the fetal lungs, breathing ceases all together, leading to 'secondary' or 'terminal apnoea'. At this point, as the fetus becomes increasingly acidotic, the heart begins to fail. If there is no effective intervention at this stage, the baby will die (in utero if unborn or ex utero if already born) and may even die despite treatment.[1] The whole process probably takes about 20 minutes in a newborn baby.[4]

While the heart continues to beat, the most important part of neonatal resuscitation is aerating the lungs. This will enable oxygenation of the heart and, hence, the brain and its respiratory centres. Unfortunately, it is not possible to tell at the time of birth whether a baby who is not breathing is in primary apnoea and about to gasp or is in the terminal apnoea phase. However, in most cases, once air enters the lungs, the infant will recover quickly and normal breathing will begin. A few babies may require cardiac massage, but usually for only a short period of time.[1]

A few babies born at the point of terminal apnoea, as mentioned previously, will die without intervention and may die despite it. In addition to ventilation and cardiac massage, drugs may be required to restore the circulation. By this stage, a senior neonatologist should be in attendance and will lead the resuscitation. If drugs are required, generally the outlook is poor for the infant.

Preparation of resuscitation equipment

Successful resuscitation is dependent on forward planning. Before any birth, it is the responsibility of the midwife and/or neonatologist to prepare and check resuscitation equipment.

It is important to check and prepare:

- clock and light
- air and suction (cylinders full and suction tubing attached)
- heater (resuscitaire) and prewarmed towels and hat
- equipment for administering air (bag/valve mask and appropriately sized mask, T-piece tubing)
- neonatal laryngoscopes (correct size blades and light working)
- notes for documentation.

When preparing for a birth, consider the woman's obstetric history and call the neonatal team and/or an additional midwife to be present in advance, if indicated. It is important to explain to the parents that a neonatologist has been called and to keep them informed of the situation.

Delayed cord clamping

The 2010 Resuscitation Council (UK) Newborn Life Support guideline recommends delayed cord clamping of at least 1 minute from the complete birth of an uncompromised infant.[1] For healthy term infants, delaying cord clamping for at least 1 minute or until the cord stops pulsating following birth improves iron status through early infancy.[1] The level at which the baby should be held in relation to the mother when delaying cord clamping in order to achieve the optimal speed and amount of placental blood transfusion is not specified in the guideline. In Andersson's study, the baby was held about 20 cm below the mother for approximately 30 seconds before placing the baby on the mother's abdomen.[5]

Taking into consideration the risk of hypothermia in the wet, newborn infant, the baby should be dried, kept warm and assessed for colour, tone, breathing and heart rate while waiting to clamp the cord.

There is currently insufficient evidence to recommend an appropriate time for clamping the cord in babies that are severely compromised at birth. Therefore, for babies requiring resuscitation, resuscitative interventions remain a priority.

Assessment and resuscitation

As with any emergency, it is important to call for help early. An outline of basic newborn resuscitation is shown in Figure 14.1, but this is not intended to be a complete guide. Further information is available from the Resuscitation Council (UK).[1,2]

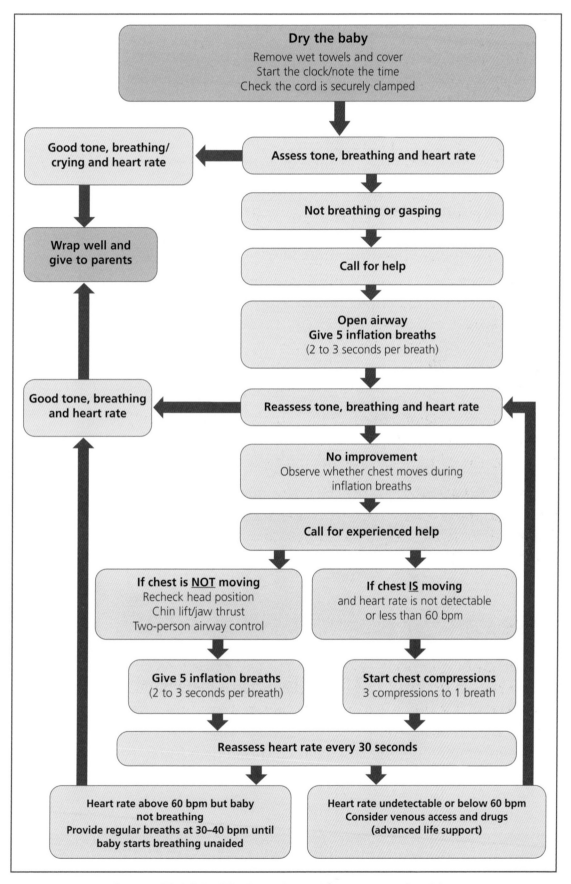

Figure 14.1 Modified newborn life support algorithm

1. Warmth and assessment at birth

Newborn babies have a large surface area to body ratio and are wet at birth. They therefore lose heat very rapidly and, if anoxic and/or small, can quickly become hypothermic.[6]

At birth:

- Start the clock and note the time of birth.

- Dry the baby, remove any wet towels and then wrap in warm dry towels, and put a hat on the baby. Drying the baby will not only stimulate the baby to breathe but will also give time for a full assessment of colour, tone, respiratory effort and heart rate (Figures 14.2 and 14.3).

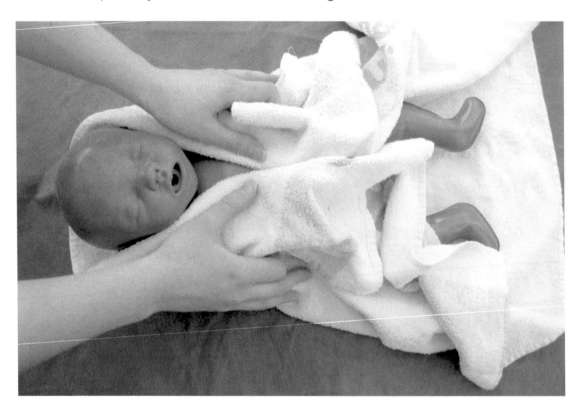

Figure 14.2 Dry the baby with a warm towel

- For uncompromised babies, delay cord clamping for at least 1 minute from the complete birth of the infant. After 1 minute, the cord should be securely clamped.

> **Resuscitative intervention remains the priority in babies who require resuscitation – do not delay cord clamping if this will interfere with neonatal resuscitation.**

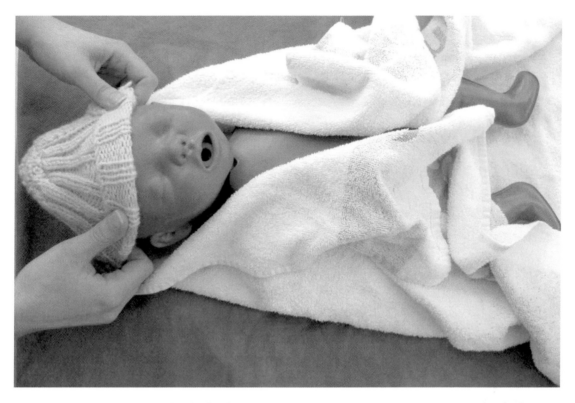

Figure 14.3 Wrap the baby in a warm dry towel and put a hat on the baby

- A healthy baby will be born blue but will have good tone, will cry within a few seconds of birth and will have a good heart rate within a few seconds of birth (the heart rate of a healthy newborn baby is about 120–150 bpm).

- A less healthy baby will be blue at birth, will have less good tone, may have a slow heart rate (less than 100 bpm) and may not establish adequate breathing by 90–120 seconds.

- An ill baby will be born pale and floppy, not breathing and with a slow, very slow or undetectable heart rate.

Preterm babies born at less than 28 weeks of gestation should be completely covered up to their necks in a food-grade plastic wrap or bag, without drying, immediately after birth (Figure 14.4). They should then be nursed under a radiant heater and stabilised. This is a very effective method of keeping preterm infants warm. They should remain wrapped until their temperature has been checked after admission to the neonatal unit. For preterm infants the labour room temperature should be at least 26°C.

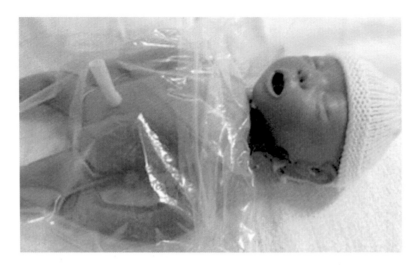

Figure 14.4 Preterm baby placed in a food bag

2. Airway

Most babies at birth have a prominent occiput which causes them to flex their neck if placed flat on their backs; this in turn blocks off their airway (Figure 14.5).

To avoid this happening, babies should be placed on their back with their head held in a neutral position (Figure 14.6). It may help to place some support under the shoulders to maintain this position.

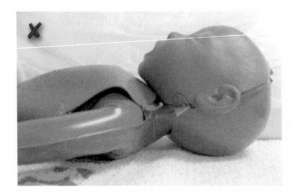

Figure 14.5 Airway obstruction caused by prominent occiput

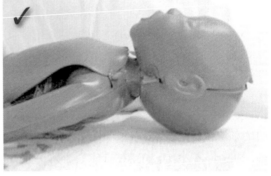

Figure 14.6 Head in the neutral position, opening the airway

If the baby is very floppy, a chin lift or jaw thrust may also be necessary to keep the airway open (Figure 14.7).

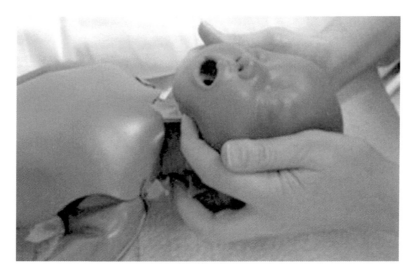

Figure 14.7 Chin lift and jaw thrust to open the airway

Airway suction immediately following birth is seldom necessary and should be reserved for babies who have obvious airway obstruction that cannot be rectified by the appropriate head positioning outlined above. Rarely, material may block the oropharynx or trachea. In these situations, direct visualisation and suction of the oropharynx should be performed. For tracheal obstruction, intubation and suction on withdrawal of the endotracheal tube may be effective but should be attempted only by an experienced practitioner.

3. Breathing

If the baby is not breathing adequately by about 90 seconds, five inflation breaths (of air) should be given. It is important that the correct size mask is used: covering the chin, but not over the eyes or squeezing the nose (Figure 14.8). The baby's lungs are filled with fluid at birth, so the inflation breaths will force out the fluid and fill the lungs with air. The pressure required to initially inflate the lungs is equivalent to 30 cm of water for 2–3 seconds/breath.[1]

If the lungs have been effectively inflated, passive movements of the chest wall will be visible and the heart rate should also increase as oxygenated blood reaches the heart. If the heart rate increases but the baby does not start breathing on his/her own, regular ventilation breaths at a rate of 30–40/minute should be continued until the baby begins to breathe for him/herself.

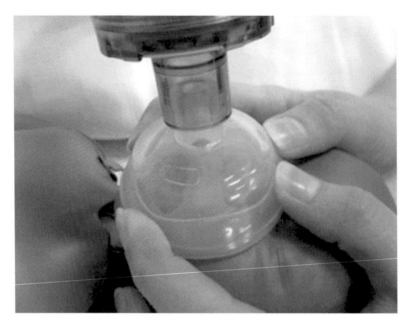

Figure 14.8 Inflation breaths using correct-sized face mask covering the nose and mouth

If the heart rate does not increase following inflation breaths, it may be because the baby needs more than lung aeration. However, the most likely cause is that the lungs have not been aerated effectively. Therefore, go back to the start and check the airway, making sure that the baby's head is in the neutral position with a jaw thrust if necessary, and that there is no obstruction in the oropharynx. If the chest wall still does not move, request assistance in maintaining the airway and consider using a Guedel airway.

If the heart rate remains slow or is absent despite five good inflation breaths with passive chest movement, chest compressions are needed and senior neonatal support should be requested.

4. Chest compression/circulation

Almost all babies needing resuscitation at birth will respond successfully to lung inflation, with a rise in heart rate proceeding rapidly to normal breathing. However, in some cases chest compression is necessary.

It is important that chest compression should only be commenced when it is certain that the lungs have been successfully inflated. Senior neonatal support should be summoned if not already in attendance.

The most efficient way to perform chest compressions in an infant is to grip the chest with both hands, with both thumbs pressing on the lower third of

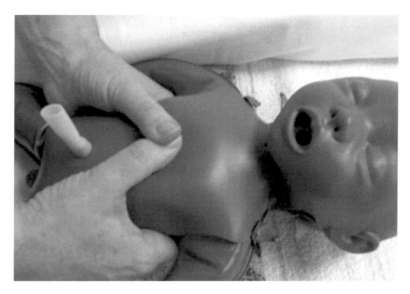

Figure 14.9 Positioning for chest compressions

the sternum, just below the nipple line, and the fingers over the spine at the back (Figure 14.9).

Compress the chest quickly and firmly to a depth of about one-third of the distance from the chest to the spine.

The ratio of compressions to breaths recommended in a newborn infant is 3:1 to achieve 90 compressions and 30 breaths in one minute.

Allow enough time between compressions for oxygenated blood to flow from the lungs to the heart at a rate of approximately 120 events/minute. Ensure that the chest is inflating with each ventilation breath.

In a very small number of babies, lung inflation and chest compressions will not be sufficient to generate an effective circulation and, in such circumstances, drugs may be required.

5. Meconium at delivery

There is no evidence that suctioning meconium from the nose and mouth of the infant while the head is still on the perineum prevents meconium aspiration, so this practice is no longer recommended.[7]

In addition, attempting to remove meconium from the airways of a vigorously crying infant has also been proved to be ineffective at preventing meconium aspiration.[8] However, if a baby is born unresponsive at birth and there is thick meconium liquor present, the oropharynx should be suctioned to clear the meconium. If intubation skills are available, the larynx and trachea should also be cleared. However, if attempted intubation is prolonged or unsuccessful, it is important to start mask ventilation, particularly if there is persistent bradycardia.

6. Emergency drugs

Emergency drugs are needed only if there is no significant circulatory response despite effective ventilation and chest compressions. A senior neonatologist should be in attendance at this stage and it is their responsibility to intubate the infant and administer medication.

7. Therapeutic hypothermia

In a newborn that is at or near term, where moderate or severe HIE is a possibility, a senior neonatologist may consider treatment with therapeutic hypothermia. If this is the case, the heater of the resuscitaire should be switched off.[1]

Documentation

It is important that all actions are documented accurately and comprehensively in the appropriate case notes, particularly when resuscitation at birth has been necessary, as records may be carefully scrutinised many years later.

References

1. Resuscitation Council (UK). *Newborn Life Support*. 3rd ed. London: Resuscitation Council (UK); 2010.

2. Resuscitation Council (UK). *Newborn Life Support: Resuscitation at Birth*. 2nd ed. London: Resuscitation Council (UK); 2006.

3. Dawes G. *Fetal and Neonatal Physiology*. Chicago: Year Book Publisher; 1968. p. 141–59.

4. Hey E, Kelly J. Gaseous exchange during endotracheal ventilation for asphyxia at birth. *J Obstet Gynaecol Br Commonw* 1968;75:414–23.

5. Andersson O, Hellström-Westas L, Andersson D, Domellöf M. Effect of delayed versus early umbilical cord clamping on neonatal outcomes and iron status at 4 months: a randomised controlled trial. *BMJ* 2011;343:d7157.

6. Dahm LS, James LS. Newborn temperature and calculated heat loss in the delivery room. *Pediatrics* 1972;49:504–13.

7. Vain NE, Szyld EG, Prudent LM, Wiswell TE, Aguilar AM, Vivas NI. Oropharyngeal and

nasopharyngeal suctioning of meconium-stained neonates before delivery of their shoulders: multicentre, randomised controlled trial. *Lancet* 2004;364:597–602.

8. Wiswell TE, Gannon CM, Jacob J, Goldsmith L, Szyld E, Weiss K, et al. Delivery room management of the apparently vigorous meconium-stained neonate: results of the multicenter, international collaborative trial. *Pediatrics* 2000;105:1–7.

Index